Monographs in the Psychology of Education

Series Editor

Daniel H. Robinson, The University of Texas at Arlington, Arlington, TX, USA

The purpose of the series, Monographs in the Psychology of Education, is to examine behavioral, cognitive, and academic assessments and interventions – with emphasis on the feasibility and reproducibility of research methods and conclusions – to determine their real-world effectiveness for students in classrooms worldwide. Series volumes provide critical reviews of evidence-based methods and may be authored or edited (multiple contributors). The books in this series serve as a critical resource for researchers, professors, and graduate students as well as clinicians, practitioners, and policy in school and clinical child psychology, special and general education, social work and all interrelated disciplines.

Hoben Thomas

Sex Differences in Reading and Math Test Scores of Children

A Heterodoxical Model

Springer

Hoben Thomas
Department of Psychology
Pennsylvania State University
University Park, PA, USA

ISSN 2662-7574 ISSN 2662-7582 (electronic)
Monographs in the Psychology of Education
ISBN 978-3-031-41271-4 ISBN 978-3-031-41272-1 (eBook)
https://doi.org/10.1007/978-3-031-41272-1

This Springer imprint is published by the registered company Springer Nature Switzerland AG
The registered company address is: Gewerbestrasse 11, 6330 Cham, Switzerland

To the love of my life, The Reverend Patricia Menné Thomas, whom I lost at the beginning of the pandemic to dementia.

Preface

Conventional wisdom is that the gender-gap or mean difference in math test scores favoring boys is negligible, vanishing, and on a path toward closure given appropriate societal adjustments. Furthermore, stereotypes and bias are the most frequently cited reasons for boys slightly larger math mean test scores. In fact, the mean gap favoring boys in math has existed since the earliest onset of achievement testing in the USA. It was evident in Stone's 1908 doctoral dissertation data and in New York City's massive math testing program in schools starting around 1910. The gap exists worldwide in most developed countries on the PISA test, as well as on the "Nation's Report Card" or NAEP tests in the USA. Of far larger size, but of nearly negligible interest, is the mean gap dramatically favoring girls in reading. In fact, girls are so dominant in reading it is difficult to find *any* studies reporting boys have larger test score means, at least in developed countries. That reading has favored girls in test score mean has been known at least since Gray's dissertation on reading tests in 1917. The convolution or finite mixture model in this book explains test score sex differences for both tasks. Interestingly, the mean differences, for both reading and math, are the *smallest* of test score sex differences. The test score variance differences, with larger variance for boys on both tasks, simply dwarf the mean differences for both tasks. The focus for more than 40 years has been on the *smaller* test score sex differences, the mean differences—arguably the wrong differences on which to focus. The theory, which is marginally more complicated than the probability model for the flip of two coins, explains these mean and variance test score differences for both tasks. The theory does so by modeling a biological mechanism which has been for decades out of favor, is nearly universally ignored, and is often disparaged. The monograph's spirit is well captured by the title of mathematician Keith Devlin's book, *The Math Gene*.

University Park, PA, USA
June 2023

Hoben Thomas

Acknowledgments

Thomas P. Hettmansperger, a long-time friend, colleague, and often coauthor is to be thanked for his help. His fingerprints are everywhere on the analytical developments. Wesley Jamison provided helpful guidance on overall organization, and especially on Chap. 1. Derek S. Young provided helpful comments as well. David R. Hunter read an early version of this work. His thoughtful comments were the basis for some rewriting and additional analysis. Finally, sincere thanks goes to Tuomas Pekkarinen, of the Helsinki School of Economics who provided means and standard deviations for the 2003 PISA scores, thereby allowing substantial additional analyses using international data. Sadly, he died in November 2022.

Contents

Chapter 1
Focus on Math and Reading Test Score Inequalities

Worldwide there has been recognition that boys' and girls' reading and math test score distributions are different. What has not been recognized is precisely how these distributions differ.

Large-scale achievement testing in the U.S. started around 1897 by J. M. Rice [1]. By 1902, the results of Rice's large-scale U.S. elementary school arithmetic reasoning tests for children were available [2]. By 1908, following C. W. Stone's efforts [3], it was clear that sixth grade boys and girls have different achievement test score distributions on each of two math tests Stone constructed. Stone's data likely provide the first evidence of sex differences in math test score distributions in the U.S.A. and perhaps globally as well. His data are typical of many other more recent examples, with small mean differences favoring boys on both tests. Figure 1.1 reveals, for the first time, data from Stone's fundamental test which shows the smaller mean difference of his two tests. Stone was surely unaware of this mean difference however and Fig. 1.1 which is a kernel density estimation plot, a graph simply unimaginable for Stone. His tools are paper and pencil. Consequently, Stone computed no quantities and no graph from these data. He likely could only stare at the tabled data on 250 boys and 250 girls he provided for each of two tests. He mused at the apparent variabilities he saw. "Doubtless the most noteworthy feature of these tables is the wide variability of achievements [3, p. 32]."

Stone's data, and Fig. 1.1 which shows that the boys' distribution is slightly right tilted relative to the girls' distribution, make clear that today's emphasis on the "gender gap," the small mean difference favoring boys in math, is nothing new. It was evident at the dawn of achievement testing, well more than 100 years ago. This fact also suggests the gap is not going away anytime soon. Early investigators may have had an inkling of such distributional differences but were unable to explicitly quantify their beliefs, which was certainly true for Stone. That distributional differences were evident at the outset of testing clearly weakens any contemporary claims that sex differences in math are the consequence of policy decisions or evolving social or environmental forces.

H. Thomas, *Sex Differences in Reading and Math Test Scores of Children*,
Monographs in the Psychology of Education,
https://doi.org/10.1007/978-3-031-41272-1_1

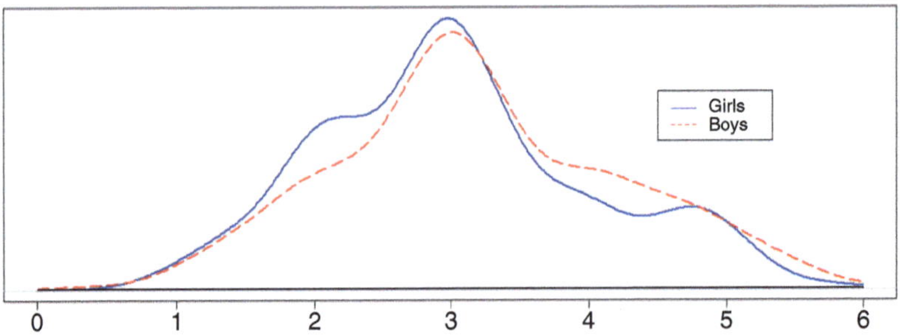

Fig. 1.1 Kernel density estimation plot of the sixth grade test scores of 250 boys and 250 girls on Stone's (1908) fundamental math test. The boys' mean is 3.193, and the girls' mean is 3.026, with corresponding standard deviations of 1.048 and 0.996

Commentary and other table entries Stone provides indicate he was well aware of sex differences in test score variability, albeit assessed with methods now obsolete and evident in small samples of his data. Also, evident in Stone's early data is a pattern of statistical features evident today in math testing studies large and small, in the U.S.A. and worldwide, patterns unrecognized by Stone—with some patterns unrecognized by investigators of sex differences in math even today. There will be more on this matter momentarily.

The situation with reading tests is similar. By 1917, Gray [4] recognized there were reading test score distributional differences between boys and girls, evident in the reading tests he constructed. But like Stone, Gray could not have appreciated the manner by which these test score distributions differed, although he did report girls' sample mean surpassed boys in oral reading in all grades one to eight of the elementary school years. Today, that girls surpass boys in reading mean is a nearly invariant universal global test result, at least in developed countries. And like the pattern of differences evident in Stone's math testing, a similar unrecognized pattern exists in reading testing data as well.

Let $\bar{x}_b$ and $\bar{x}_g$ denote test score sample means of boys and girls, respectively, with s_b^2 and s_g^2 their corresponding sample variances. The way sex differences are defined today is by effect size d with

$$d = \frac{\bar{x}_b - \bar{x}_g}{\sqrt{(s_b^2 + s_g^2)/2}}.$$

While d can be viewed as an empirical method of gauging sex differences, most of the writers treat it as an inferential quantity, in which case the appropriateness of d's use rests on the probability model for d or δ,

$$\delta = \frac{\mu_b - \mu_g}{\sigma_c},$$

and μ_b and μ_g are the population means for boys and girls, respectively. σ_c is the assumed common population standard deviation. So d presumably estimates δ.

Although there has been no conceptual defense arguing that d is the most appropriate scalar index for behavioral sex differences data, d has nonetheless been for decades the nearly sole unquestioned index by which sex differences on a myriad of variables have been assessed in journal articles, meta-analyses, and books [5, 6].

However, d has led nowhere. It has provided no assistance in understanding the origins of sex differences in reading or math or why they persist. Worse, outcomes of d meta-analyses are often puzzling. A common math finding is that the mean d, that is, $\bar{d}$, is positive but small and favors boys. For example, in Lakin [7], the overall math $\bar{d} = 0.077$. Why these small (scaled) mean differences appear has befuddled investigators [8–10].

Meanwhile, it has long been recognized that typically

$$s_b > s_g \text{ or } s_b^2/s_g^2 > 1$$

holds for both tasks, reading and math. These inequalities have also long perplexed researchers [9, 11–14].

Writers and those with a penchant for d-based meta-analyses, as well as many researchers, have slavishly, seemingly lemminglike, taken d as the ultimate sex differences scalar index. It has even been claimed d is useful for *any* sex differences variable [15, p. 177]. δ, the model for d, is conceptually inappropriate as the need to report s_b^2/s_g^2 implicitly makes clear. More importantly, d is a misleading way of viewing sex differences, at least for math and reading test score data. That is because d has directed attention toward mean differences and misdirected attention away from the *far larger* variance differences in data. Once these differences are properly recognized, one is forced to recognize the inadequacies of d. More centrally however, it forces a need to rethink how differences between the sexes should be viewed, again at least for reading and math test score data.

The key for understanding is not to focus on scaled sample mean differences, as d requires. Rather, focus instead on summary data statistical *inequalities*. In particular, focus on pairs of inequalities. These are the data patterns that must be explained by any creditable framework which is claimed to account for sex differences in math and reading.

Define the following two sets, the inequalities of which may appear familiar, first for math testing and then reading testing, respectively:

$$mo = \{\bar{x}_b > \bar{x}_g \;\&\; s_b > s_g\} \text{ and}$$

$$ro = \{\bar{x}_g > \bar{x}_b \;\&\; s_b > s_g\}.$$

The inequalities of the following two sets have apparently never before been recognized. Again, the first set is for math testing the second set is for reading testing:

$$mdo = \{s_b^2 - s_g^2 > \bar{x}_b - \bar{x}_g, \text{given } mo\} \text{ and}$$

$$rdo = \{s_b^2 - s_g^2 > \bar{x}_g - \bar{x}_b, \text{given } ro\}.$$

Call these four sets collectively,

$$\mathcal{S} = \{mo, ro, mdo, rdo\}.$$

Read mo as "math order," ro as "reading order," mdo as "math difference order," and rdo as "reading difference order." The primary task of this monograph can be easily stated: model the data structures of $\mathcal{S}$.

One's intuition with numbers can often lead one astray, regardless of how technically skilled one might be [16], and there may be repeated instances in the following pages when this may be the case. So, consider

$$\bar{x}_b = 152, \bar{x}_g = 149, s_b = 34 + 3, s_g = 34.$$

Relative sizes are easy numerical comparisons, so it is easily seen in this math test example that mo is satisfied. However, mdo may seem not only a strange comparison but intuitively more challenging as well. One easily observes the difference $s_b - s_g = 3$ which might seem small. But the required difference to consider is $s_b^2 - s_g^2 = 213$, which perhaps seems larger than intuitively expected and far larger than $\bar{x}_b - \bar{x}_g$. Small differences in standard deviations can balloon into large differences in variance. There is not a unique way of thinking about the matter, but the numerical values of s_b and s_g above were written in the form $w + b$ and w, respectively, a difference independent of w. The variance difference $(w + b)^2 - w^2 = b^2 + 2bw$ increases quadratically in b or linearly in w, so the example provides perhaps an "intuitive correction" going forward. The example is from Table 2.3, Chap. 2, "The Nation's Report Card" 12th grade 2019 math testing result.

Although it was claimed decades ago that the sex mean differences on cognitive tests were disappearing [17], or at least in more recent decades that the mean sex differences in math have decreased [18], or that the test gaps in math mean are "...close to zero in developed countries...[19, p. 1219]," keeping alive perhaps the hope that the small mean sex difference favoring boys in math test scores will soon vanish with suitable societal changes. This hope is simply wishful thinking. The empirical fact remains that, from the perspective of more than a century, the inequalities of $\mathcal{S}$ have widely held, and they continue to do so worldwide, in developed countries, with an occasional exception, but only for math. Furthermore, the mean gap is not even the largest sex differences gap as $\mathcal{S}$ makes clear. Moreover, at least in the U.S.A., the small math mean difference disadvantaging girls has garnered nearly all the attention. By contrast, girls' mean advantage in reading is *multiples larger* than boys' mean advantage in math. Yet by comparison, the interest in sex differences in reading has been little more than a footnote.

The inequalities of $\mathcal{S}$ are so ubiquitous in the literature, as will be demonstrated in Chap. 2, they may be said to *characterize* the structure of the literature for children's reading and math test score summary statistics. The data for Stone's fundamental test displayed in Fig. 1.1 satisfies mo. His reasoning test satisfies mdo. The inequalities of $\mathcal{S}$ are the focus of sex differences throughout. Importantly, they tightly constrain the class of models that accounts for them in a coherent way. Happily, as it turns out, accounting for these inequalities also provides the basis for explaining other widely recognized empirical facts long unaccounted for in the reading and math observational test score sex differences literature.

This monograph has four main goals:

1. To demonstrate the ubiquity of inequalities of $\mathcal{S}$ in the broad *observational* child math and reading achievement test score literature.
2. To provide a coherent model that accounts for the inequalities of $\mathcal{S}$.
3. To provide coherent accounts for other well-recognized yet unexplained empirical differences in boys' and girls' reading and math test score distributions. As an example, an issue of wide-spread puzzlement in math testing concerns the right tails of boys' and girls' test score distributions. The right tail for boys typically has a larger empirical data mass than the corresponding right tail for girls. Stone's data in Fig. 1.1 provide suggestive evidence for this widely recognized empirical fact. Less well recognized is that focusing on the left tails of the reading test score distributions reveals boys have a larger empirical data mass than do girls. So, boys share an unexplained "infamy" for their anchoring of the tails of distributions associated with tasks arguably representing the most important skills children will ever need.

   Indeed, boys are far more overrepresented in the bottom of the reading test distribution than they are overrepresented in the top part of the math test distribution, as will be seen later. The goal is to address these puzzles in a coherent way within a suitable model.
4. The final goal is to provide model parameter estimates, thus illuminating, with numerous associated graphics, the model's plausibility.

While the focus here is narrow and confined, namely the reading and math *observational* test score literature, that literature is substantial. It includes reported test standardization data, large sample surveys, and observational studies of children's test scores obtained in classroom settings. That girls achieve higher grades than boys in the classroom, a success that does not seem to translate to other settings is a well-recognized and important fact [20]. However, it is an example of a matter that is outside the neighborhood of focus here.

Efforts to address sex differences, especially in math, nearly always cast a far larger net. For Ceci and Williams, 2010 [5], test score differences are only a small part of their far larger agenda. Their primary focus is why there are relatively few women in engineering, computer science, and other math-oriented occupations. These issues are certainly compelling but are not addressed here. However, some findings from the present analysis seem to have relevance for understanding sex differences observed in larger social contexts. When this is recognized, the possible implications will be noted.

The path taken here is different and likely to be unfamiliar. The literature on sex differences is dominated by conventional statistical approaches featuring regressions, correlational analyses, path diagrams, and effect sizes. No conventional statistical approaches are featured here. This announcement should not surprise. That is because no conventional approach has been able to coherently explain the inequalities of concern nor the many perplexing empirical facts of data. The evidence is clear: after decades of attention, there has been no compelling explanation, using a myriad of conventional statistical approaches, why the most fixated feature of attention, which has essentially defined interest in sex differences in math, the mean gender gap, exists or why it persists. Furthermore, the task is more complex than explaining the mean difference, the focus of nearly all research. The much larger variance differences must be addressed as well. And this goal must be achieved not just for math sex differences but also for reading sex differences.

Consequently, a new framework must be provided. It is developed below. That new framework is a probability model called model $\mathcal{Y}$. It is developed in Chap. 4 and is the framework within which all sex differences in test score distributions are viewed. The model forms the only basis for interpretation of sex differences throughout. In addition, of course, $\mathcal{Y}$ requires a new parameter estimation or statistical procedure which is provided. One feature of the approach is that there is no appeal to covariates as is commonly the case. Covariates may be important, but they play no role in the analyses that follow.

In addition, the path forward is likely to be, for some readers at least, unpopular. It would certainly be preferable if this were not the case. However, to explain test score sex differences coherently, there appears no choice: a genetical theory of X-linkage appears to be the only viable perspective available, and when suitably modeled, it is remarkably parsimonious. It requires just three parameters, the same number as δ, so it might be hoped readers can warm to the idea. Such an idea was decades ago mocked or ignored, an attitude that persists today, at least in some quarters. However, a model so based accounts remarkably well for the sex differences observed, as well as the inequalities. To anticipate matters, the empirical inequalities of $\mathcal{S}$ are just *expectations* under the model proposed.

Genetical models have never been widely popular, at least in most psychological circles, and their role in explaining behaviors is often grudgingly acknowledged if acknowledged at all. However, it is important to recognize that genetical models have never been proposed to explain behaviors when other coherent explanations were available. As Ceci and Williams 2010 note, advances in understanding "...comes from free and open debate in which all sides present their best evidence and no one is excoriated for arguing the unpopular side [5, p. 219]."

This plea for openness was expressed more than a decade ago. Is the current psychological science environment open to unpopular perspectives? Staddon [21] certainly does not think so. He castigates individuals, universities, funding institutions, and more for their lack of openness in science to ideas and intellectual diversity. Staddon compares the current situation, especially with respect to understanding group cognitive differences, with Lysenkoism [21, p. 167]. In fact, the spirit of Lysenkoism is now seen as threatening *all of science* [22].

Can one, nonetheless, expect a spirit of openness to ideas and conceptualizations regarding unexplained sex differences in reading and math test scores? One certainly hopes so especially for what follows here. But the overall outlook appears cloudy at best if the path forward is to report only the most austere empirical facts. An example is a recent article which reports sex differences associated with the most innocuous, banal, everyday adult behaviors, such as cooking, sewing on a button, or washing cars [23]. Yet it is written in a remarkably cautious style. Just how *to refer* to sex differences requires, for the authors, a definition: "...we label differences by the hybrid neologisms of gender/sex...and sex/gender...and apply these terms interchangeably [23, p. 1340]." They strive to avoid any scintilla that would suggest mechanisms producing such differences by stressing "...we assiduously avoid discussing particular causal explanations of gender/sex differences and similarities or indicating our personal preferences for any theories of causation [23, p. 1340])." And some readers may view their discussion as seeming to apologize for even pointing out that there *are* sex differences, perhaps fearing they might antagonize some readers (in particular, journal editors). They write near their close "...our insights that sex/gender differences can be simultaneously large and small might appear to some readers to threaten gender equality [23, p. 1354]." Should this last quote be understood to mean simply recognizing that to "cook meat on the grill" is a more masculine than feminine task is likely to pose a threat to gender equality? One can guess at the ramifications for the study of sex differences should this writing style become the template for the future. It would surely curtail a core goal of the scientific process, causal explanations, or as Judea Pearl would put it: Why? [24].

Doubtlessly, anyone who has studied the sex differences literature has observed the inequality pairs in mo and ro. They are simply too dominant in the literature to avoid notice. The surprise is that the mdo and rdo inequalities widely hold. In fact, the size of the sample variance differences usually *far* exceeds the sample mean differences. It is difficult to imagine any other fact of empirical data that would signal a more robust rejection of conventional perspectives on how sex differences are viewed, namely that mean differences capture the essence of distributional differences, at least for math and reading sex differences test scores. These empirical facts, to be surveyed in Chap. 2, would seem to provide overwhelming conceptual problems for those who claim the sex differences in math are vanishing, ignorable, or may not exist at all [25].

Small sex differences, in sample means, especially in math, have enjoyed the attention while variance differences have largely been ignored, or at least from a substantive perspective, discounted. The reasons for this emphasis on means and not variances are not difficult to discern and involve both technical and psychological considerations. One psychological reason is that it is easy to *think* in terms of group differences as simply realizations of visual images likely to be familiar: two identically shaped typically normal-like or "bell-shaped" distributions shifted slightly apart, consequently differing only in mean. This is an example of what are termed *location-shift* models; the intuition is compelling. δ is a scaled version of a location-shift model. Where variances and their differences are concerned, these intuitive advantages seem to disappear.

The dominance of effect size d as a sex difference defining assessment tool has certainly reinforced this mean difference perspective. Of course, the widely used expression "gender gap" reinforces this cognitive perspective. Sometimes variance parameters are called *nuisance parameters* [26, p. 3] signaling the perceived unimportance of variances. The most commonly used statistical models often assume equal population variances, with a corresponding central attention on population means. Analytically unequal population variances have been historically troublesome for statistical theory and consequently applied researchers as well. Some of these issues seem practically unimportant now with computing replacing analysis, as with the bootstrap [27].

Still, thinking intuitively about the mechanisms that might produce variance differences in behavior seems cognitively difficult. Yet sample variance differences are by far the dominate feature of reading and math test score sex difference summary statistics. This is the reality, and this reality has been unchanged for decades. To repeat, any sex differences theory must account for variance differences and the mean differences as well. This fact was recognized by Feingold in 1992 [28] who argued, correctly, that to understand cognitive sex differences both means and variances must *jointly* be considered. But efforts to do so have not subsequently appeared.

Now, fully 30 years later appears an article with title "Joint Consideration of Means and Variances Might Change the Understanding of Etiology" [29]. The article is a welcome addition. But it focuses largely on adoption or twin studies within the context of conventional behavioral genetics approaches and does not consider its larger conceptual importance. No new framework is proposed. The place to start is at the model level and perhaps with discrete probability models. That is because in all popular ones, the binomial, negative binomial, Poisson, and geometric, the means and variances are linked through their shared common parameters. Instead, the authors focus at the data analysis level.

The literature review will consider only readily accessible reading and math observational test score literature and focuses on whether the inequalities of $\mathcal{S}$ are satisfied or not. Thus, mostly reported are studies which report the key quantities of focus, the sample means, and sample variances (or standard deviations) for both boys and girls. These statistics will be denoted by V defined by

$$V = \{\bar{x}_b, \bar{x}_g, s_b, s_g\}.$$

If sample sizes are also available, V will appear with six elements

$$V = \{\bar{x}_b, \bar{x}_g, s_b, s_g, n_b, n_g\},$$

where n_b and n_g are boys' and girls' sample sizes, respectively.

In all that follows, V are the only data of focus. No new data are reported. Unless V is explicitly reported, mdo and rdo cannot be evaluated. If mdo holds or rdo holds, then mo or ro must hold as well. However, mo or ro can hold while the more constraining inequalities of differences, mdo or rdo, can fail. They can fail simply because of the noise of real data, and probabilistically, they are more likely to do so. Sometimes reported are d and s_b^2/s_g^2, which enables mo or ro to be evaluated, but without being able to explicitly define the elements of V, in which case mdo or rdo cannot be evaluated.

Thus, the thrust of the literature review is to illustrate the dominance of the inequalities in several domains. This perspective departs sharply from the current practice which defaults to d as the sex difference index, which is often coupled with the belief that small d, however consistently signed, or that ratios of s_b^2/s_g^2 however consistently greater than one, are apparently ignorable.

In fact, the consistency of mo and ro in the observational math and reading test score literature must stand as one of the most remarkably consistent and easily observable empirical findings in the child literature. And the evidence has been but a mouse click away. To anticipate, simply glance at the "Nation's Report Card" data [30] reproduced in Table 2.1 through Table 2.4 in Chap. 2. That mo or ro widely hold is immediately evident. Less obvious is that the inequalities of rdo and mdo nearly always hold as well. These results are based on millions of children assessed over decades using evolving but remarkably sophisticated and representative research protocols.

There has long been a dismissive attitude toward small differences in sample values, especially sample means. For example, Miller and Halpern write "Sex differences in average mathematics test performance also decreased during the 1970s to 1980s and have since remained small to *negligible* [18, p. 38, italics added]." In fact, they go further explicitly *defining* cognitive sex differences as mean differences, so variance differences are apparently irrelevant. One would expect s_b^2/s_g^2 to fluctuate about one, if δ, the model for d, were appropriate. Additionally, one would expect d to fluctuate about zero if boys and girls followed the same test score distribution. In fact, neither is the case. Miller and Halpern [18] reference Lakin [7] to support their claim. Lakin reported data implying 28 V. Of these, 26 satisfied mo. Thus, all but two implied V satisfied both $\bar{x}_b > \bar{x}_g$ and $s_b > s_g$. Furthermore, Lakin employed CogAT test standardization data with huge sample sizes and data spanning decades.

A dramatic example of $s_b^2/s_g^2 > 1$ consistency was dispatched as unimportant. It appears in *Science*, where a green colored headline proclaims: "Standardized tests in the U.S. indicate girls now score just as well as boys in math [9, p. 494]." The data source is state math test data from 10 U.S. states. In Table S1 [31] are reported d, variance ratios, and sample sizes, data equivalent to 66 V. The sample sizes are typically in the tens to hundreds of thousands. Of the 66 variance ratios, 65 satisfy $s_b^2/s_g^2 > 1$. This fact was noted but dismissed with the observation: "However, none are very large and... the male variance is not markedly greater than female variance [31, p. 2]." Such remarkable consistencies need an explanation, not dismissal.

Much more variables were the 66 d which range from -0.13 to 0.10, with $\bar{d} = -.007$ a rare negative value computed from data in their Table S1. However, how the tests vary from state to state and their corresponding content appears unknown. It is only on math tests with a reasoning component that boys display a typically small mean advantage. This will be clear in Chap. 2. These data also speak to the consistency with which the variance differences, $s_b^2 - s_g^2$ are often more consistently positive (or equivalently, $s_b^2/s_g^2 > 1$), while the mean differences $\bar{x}_b - \bar{x}_g$ often seem more apt to fluctuate in sign—but only for math: for reading, $\bar{x}_b - \bar{x}_g > 0$ essentially never appears.

The perspective here is that it is the *consistency* of the outcomes over realizations of V that is far more important than the sizes of the mean differences within V which, only for math, and not reading, are often small. This attitude contrasts sharply with some other perspectives and attitudes toward regularities in empirical data. An example concerns d or $\bar{d}$, which, as noted earlier, has persistently been observed in math meta-analyses to be positive but small, favoring boys. This empirical fact apparently has been an irritation. A "solution" has been proposed: simply *define* the problem away! Hyde and colleagues have long defined $d \leq 0.10$ as *trivial* [9, 15, 25, 32] (The definition probably intended is $|d| \leq 0.10$.) or alternatively as "...an effect so small as to be considered no gender difference [33, p. 8801]." A conceptual explanation of why small $d > 0$ persistently appears in math studies and corresponding $\bar{d} > 0$ in meta-analyses will be provided later in Chap. 6.

Kagan in 2012 viewed psychological research as in crisis and suggested several reforms researchers should take to fix the matter. Kagan writes: "The most important reform urges a search for patterns in the body of evidence... [34, p. 249]." The thrust here is very much in this spirit. A goal of the literature review is to establish the consistency of the patterns of inequalities of $\mathcal{S}$ over several domains, including children's ages, countries, tests, and time frames.

Following the literature review in Chap. 2 and a chapter on alternative perspectives in Chap. 3, the theory will be developed in Chap. 4. As noted, it will be revealed that the inequalities of $\mathcal{S}$ are simply expectations under the theory proposed. Consequently, the data inequalities are nothing surprising. Subsequently, in Chap. 5, many math and reading V examples will be analyzed, their parameter estimates given, with many solutions graphically portrayed. Chapter 6 summarizes matters, extends the analysis in some ways, and applies the model framework to selected settings.

Transparency and Openness (TOP): all analytical results, estimation procedures, and computer code are contained herein or are in Appendix A. All V which have been identified, which are publicly available and readily accessible, form the basis for the review in Chap. 2. It would appear that the research reported here satisfies TOP level three criteria for all eight standards, where applicable [35].

Chapter 2
Literature Review with Focus on Inequalities

Evidence of the inequalities of S come from several sources. They are widely evident in large scale U.S. national and international PISA studies, which provide compelling evidence. Numerous other studies including the earliest U.S. achievement tests also provide similar evidence.

2.1 U.S. National and International Studies

2.1.1 NAEP: "The Nation's Report Card"

U.S. reading and math data are available from the largest most representative and congressionally mandated U.S. assessment, the National Assessment of Educational Progress (NAEP), known as the "Nation's Report Card" [30]. From NAEP's 1969 start when in the early days John Tukey was technical advisor, it has evolved both technically and legislatively. Millions of children have been assessed over the years, with from 10,000 to 20,000 children involved in nationwide grade level assessment [36]. There can be little doubt that NAEP tests are by far the best estimates of children's math and reading achievements for the U.S.A. and thus correspondingly information on sex differences as well. The NAEP tests have been called the "gold standard" for monitoring children's academic progress [37, p. vii]. However, the estimates provided are not conventional simple random sample estimates nor do they possess random sample estimate properties.

The NAEP sampling procedure is multistage, clustered, and stratified. First, the U.S.A. is partitioned into primary sampling units (PSUs) which involve one or more counties, and then there is sampling of schools within the PSU and then students within schools. About 30 children are tested within sampled schools [38] with each tested child receiving a *random sample* of test items, in one of many different test

H. Thomas, *Sex Differences in Reading and Math Test Scores of Children*,
Monographs in the Psychology of Education,
https://doi.org/10.1007/978-3-031-41272-1_2

booklets [26, Chapter 2]. Thus, no child receives more than a very small sample of items, and estimates of individual children are not possible, but groups of children can be compared. Coupled with the NAEP complex sampling procedure is the estimation procedure involving Item Response Theory, latent variables, multiple imputation, numerical integration, student weights, and more [26, 37, 39]. A further consequence is that sample sizes are not meaningfully associated with estimated quantities.

The most elementary generally recognized necessary requirement of any statistical estimate is that it is *consistent.* That is, one "does better" as sample size increases, so the sample estimates approach their parameter values as sample sizes increase. The consistency of the estimates in NAEP-like settings is not assured [26, p. 29]. This fact is made intuitively plausible at the individual subject level because each child is given only a few of the possible test items available. Consequently, the consistency of an estimate of a child's ability may not be achieved, a fact that can have implications in subsequent procedures. For the NAEP estimated means and standard deviations, standard errors are not reported. Their calculation, usually involving *jackknifing*, is not straightforward given the complexity of the sampling and estimate procedures [39].

These details concerning the NAEP sampling and estimation procedures make it abundantly clear that conventional textbook statistical tools useful for random samples are simply inappropriate. However, some other investigators have, nevertheless, forged ahead with standard statistical procedures [40].

These same general procedures employed in the NAEP surveys are employed in the international surveys, such as the PISA tests, noted below, which were modeled after the NAEP procedures. And these facts have further implications for estimates *based* on V estimates from large sample survey procedures. It means, as is noted subsequently, that there is no guidance for the construction of standard errors of parameter estimates based on V from large sample surveys.

Tables 2.1 and 2.2 display NAEP math and reading means and standard deviations at Grades 4 and 8. Tables 2.3 and 2.4 display math and reading at Grade 12 [30]. The columns of these tables are labeled $\bar{x}_b$, $\bar{x}_g$, s_b, and s_g. This notation is for consistency only; they are not conventional sample means and standard deviations for reasons just addressed. In these tables, those V which fail to satisfy either mo or ro appear in bold font. Otherwise, all V satisfy the stronger order relation, mdo or rdo. In Table 2.1, of 26 V for math, 23 satisfy mdo, while 23 of 27 reading V satisfy rdo in Table 2.2. Similarly, Tables 2.3 and 2.4 display twelfth grade math and reading data. For twelfth grade reading, seven of eight V satisfy rdo. All five math V satisfy mdo. Collectively, of the 66 NAEP V, in these tables 58 or all but 8 satisfy mdo or rdo. Seven of the eight failures are ties, likely the result of rounding.

The mean differences in math are always small. The boys' mean never exceeds the mean of the girls by more than three points, but it is the consistency, spanning decades, which is striking. While the mean differences in math are always small, the mean differences in reading favoring girls are substantially larger, and girls *always* have larger means. The girls' mean reading advantage ranges from 6 to 15 points, and girls never show less than a 9-point mean advantage at the eighth and twelfth

Table 2.1 NAEP Grades 4 and 8 Math

	4th				8th			
Year	$\bar{x}_b$	$\bar{x}_g$	s_b	s_g	$\bar{x}_b$	$\bar{x}_g$	s_b	s_g
2019	242	239	33	30	**282**	**282**	40	38
2017	241	239	33	30	283	282	40	38
2015	241	239	31	29	**282**	**282**	38	36
2013	242	241	30	29	285	284	38	35
2011	241	240	30	28	284	283	37	35
2009	241	239	30	28	284	282	37	35
2007	241	239	29	28	282	280	37	35
2005	239	237	29	28	280	278	37	35
2003	236	233	29	28	278	277	37	35
2000	227	224	32	30	274	272	38	36
1996	224	223	32	30	271	269	38	37
1992	221	219	33	31	**268**	**269**	37	36
1990	214	213	33	31	263	262	37	35

Note: Bold font denotes mo failure

Table 2.2 NAEP Grades 4 and 8 Reading

	4th				8th			
Year	$\bar{x}_b$	$\bar{x}_g$	s_b	s_g	$\bar{x}_b$	$\bar{x}_g$	s_b	s_g
2019	217	224	39	37	258	269	38	36
2017	219	225	39	37	262	272	36	35
2015	219	226	38	37	261	270	35	34
2013	219	225	38	36	263	273	**34**	**34**
2011	218	225	37	35	261	270	35	33
2009	218	224	36	34	259	269	35	33
2007	218	224	36	35	258	268	35	34
2005	216	222	**36**	**36**	257	267	35	34
2003	215	222	38	36	258	269	36	34
2002	215	222	**36**	**36**	260	269	34	33
2000	208	219	42	40	NA	NA	NA	NA
1998	212	217	**39**	**39**	256	270	36	33
1994	209	220	42	39	252	267	37	35
1992	213	221	36	34	254	267	36	35

Note: Bold font denotes ro failure. NA = not available

Table 2.3 NAEP Grade 12 Math

Year	$\bar{x}_b$	$\bar{x}_g$	s_b	s_g
2019	152	149	37	34
2015	153	150	35	33
2013	155	152	34	32
2009	155	152	35	32
2005	151	149	36	32

Note: All V satisfy mdo

Table 2.4 NAEP Grade 12 Reading

Year	$\bar{x}_b$	$\bar{x}_g$	s_b	s_g
2015	282	292	41	39
2013	284	293	39	36
2009	282	294	39	36
2005	279	292	39	37
2002	279	295	37	36
1998	285	298	38	35
1994	280	294	**36**	**36**
1992	282	297	33	32

Note: Bold font denotes *ro* failure

grade levels. Of those V satisfying mdo, the median ratio of $(s_b^2 - s_g^2)/(\bar{x}_b - \bar{x}_g)$ is 72, so the variance differences dwarf the mean differences. The median of the corresponding rdo reading ratio $(s_b^2 - s_g^2)/(\bar{x}_g - \bar{x}_b)$ is 13. In summary, mdo and rdo widely hold in the NAEP reading and math data. The story is little changed in other settings.

2.1.2 PISA Tests

The 2015 Programme for International Student Assessment (PISA) tests [41, 42], which involve 5000 students from each country, reveal that for those 15 to 16 year olds, girls' reading average exceeded boys' average in all 44 countries, averaging 27 points. Among 42 countries with math data, boys' average exceeded the girls' average in 35 countries by 8 points. Variances are not easily accessible for the 2015 data.

Tables 2.5 and 2.6 display the PISA means and standard deviations for math and reading for 41 countries in the 2003 testing cycle [43, 44]. While these published reports do not contain means and standard deviations for each country, they were graciously provided by Tuomas Pekkarinen, of the Helsinki School of Economics. Again, these means and standard deviations are not conventional sample estimates, although the column labels use familiar notation. In Table 2.5 mdo holds for 36 of 41 countries; for the five countries shown in bold font, mo fails. In Table 2.6, all 41 reading V satisfy rdo.

As with the NAEP data, the sizes of the boys math mean exceeding the girls math mean are far smaller than for the corresponding reading differences favoring girls. The 39 positive $\bar{x}_b - \bar{x}_g$ math differences ranged from 1.21 to 28.84 with mean difference 11.34. For reading, all $\bar{x}_g - \bar{x}_b$ were positive, with differences ranging from 13.27 to 57.76 and mean difference 33.63. Clearly, girls dominate boys in every OECD country in reading at least in 2015 and 2003.

Table 2.5 PISA Math 2003

Country	$\bar{x}_b$	$\bar{x}_g$	s_b	s_g
Australia	526.89	521.55	99.23	91.25
Austria	509.39	501.82	97.12	88.74
Belgium	532.88	525.37	114.35	104.69
Brazil	364.70	348.44	104.18	95.10
Canada	540.77	529.60	92.16	82.89
Czech Republic	523.84	508.87	97.32	93.94
Denmark	522.73	506.15	90.77	91.15
Finland	548.00	540.60	87.63	79.41
France	515.28	506.76	95.68	87.80
Germany	507.87	498.90	105.07	99.31
Greece	454.95	435.55	98.13	88.65
Hong Kong	552.40	548.35	107.44	92.30
Hungary	493.70	485.90	95.46	91.15
Iceland	507.65	523.06	94.55	85.01
Indonesia	361.84	358.50	79.35	81.61
Ireland	510.18	495.38	86.32	83.55
Italy	474.92	457.09	100.97	89.69
Japan	538.53	530.11	106.74	94.14
Korea	551.71	528.31	93.35	89.17
Latvia	484.84	482.03	91.77	84.18
Lichtenstein	549.84	521.00	105.68	89.83
Luxembourg	501.93	484.76	94.77	88.16
Macau-China	538.19	516.94	91.32	81.38
Mexico	390.87	379.97	87.04	83.60
Netherlands	540.33	535.22	92.39	92.62
New Zealand	530.71	516.23	101.51	94.45
Norway	498.27	492.05	95.96	87.79
Poland	493.04	487.45	95.50	84.63
Portugal	472.44	460.19	93.23	81.82
Russian Federation	473.50	463.38	96.30	87.82
Slovakia	507.29	488.63	94.94	90.61
Serbia	437.48	436.27	90.14	78.94
Spain	489.61	480.74	92.28	84.41
Sweden	512.31	505.78	96.86	92.50
Switzerland	534.58	517.95	100.40	95.45
Thailand	414.77	418.79	84.16	80.08
Tunisia	364.91	352.74	82.31	81.23
Turkey	430.23	415.09	109.00	98.68
United Kingdom	511.80	505.14	93.66	90.92
United States	485.96	479.71	99.15	91.03
Uruguay	428.39	416.30	102.01	97.07

Note: mo fails for countries in bold font. 36 countries satisfy mdo

Table 2.6 PISA Reading 2003

Country	$\bar{x}_b$	$\bar{x}_g$	s_b	s_g
Australia	506.09	545.43	100.47	89.81
Austria	467.13	514.35	105.46	94.91
Belgium	489.33	526.23	113.55	102.58
Brazil	384.22	418.85	115.85	104.57
Canada	514.00	545.53	92.77	82.58
Czech Republic	473.10	504.40	95.36	93.05
Denmark	479.39	504.80	89.77	85.03
Finland	521.39	565.41	82.43	73.34
France	476.10	514.29	99.99	90.50
Germany	470.80	512.93	111.45	102.20
Greece	452.88	490.37	110.19	95.54
Hong Kong	493.83	525.36	90.67	75.26
Hungary	467.24	498.20	92.93	88.12
Iceland	463.81	521.57	99.92	87.25
Indonesia	369.48	393.52	75.43	75.27
Ireland	501.08	530.10	87.08	83.51
Italy	455.24	494.59	105.42	92.23
Japan	486.57	508.98	110.70	99.11
Korea	525.48	546.73	83.38	79.77
Latvia	470.40	509.14	93.23	83.50
Lichtenstein	516.60	534.00	93.19	85.70
Luxembourg	462.66	495.66	103.3	93.22
Macau-China	490.82	504.09	69.41	63.92
Mexico	388.59	410.07	96.23	92.93
Netherlands	502.87	523.78	85.70	82.63
New Zealand	507.73	535.35	107.14	100.20
Norway	475.34	524.54	105.07	93.48
Poland	476.78	516.33	99.65	87.77
Portugal	458.52	494.86	97.24	84.84
Russian Federation	427.84	456.36	97.68	86.39
Serbia	389.93	433.05	83.29	73.70
Slovakia	453.28	485.82	92.71	89.36
Spain	460.66	499.78	98.65	88.08
Sweden	495.91	532.66	96.22	91.39
Switzerland	481.99	517.49	96.22	89.76
Thailand	396.45	439.17	78.35	72.48
Tunisia	361.77	387.10	95.22	94.63
Turkey	425.97	459.31	98.85	87.25
United Kingdom	491.82	520.37	95.86	90.20
United States	479.29	511.30	103.82	95.80
Uruguay	414.02	453.32	125.44	114.40

Note: All 41 countries satisfy *rdo*

2.1.3 IEA PIRLS and TIMSS Tests

The International Association for the Evaluation of Educational Achievement (IEA) sponsors the Progress in International Reading Literacy Study or PIRLS test which assesses reading among fourth graders and the Trends in International Mathematics and Science Study or TIMSS math tests which assess fourth and eighth graders as well as a more advanced TIMSS-advanced math test administered in the last year of secondary school. Among 79 *V*, mostly different countries in the 2001 and 2006 PIRLS reading assessments [14], 62 satisfied *rdo*. Never did the boys' mean exceed the girls' mean in reading. Among 55 countries and 55 *V* in 2015 TIMSS fourth graders math test, 32 of 55 satisfied *mdo*; for the 2015 TIMSS eighth graders, among 46 *V* 19 satisfied *mdo*, while among 10 counties in the 2015 TIMMS-advanced math, 7 satisfied *mdo* [45]. The TIMSS fourth and eighth grade tests but perhaps not on the advanced test reveal outcome patterns relatively different from those for NAEP or PISA tests, and the reason seems to be the content of the tests. It is generally understood that the TIMSS items assess more basic skills than do the PISA and NAEP math tests [46] and thus are correspondingly less comparable to them. As will be noted shortly, it has been known for a century from large sample New York City school data, girls exceed boys on some arithmetic tests in grade school and high school.

2.2 Publicly Accessible Individual Studies Reporting *V*

Six thousand entering students in 47 California junior colleges received the math portion of the Iowa High School test during the 1929–1930 class year. *mdo* holds [47]. Of 21 *V* 19 satisfy *ro*, and among these 19, 17 also satisfy *rdo* for seven grades and three reading tests [48]. Among a combined third grade sample, *rdo* holds [49]. For 10-year old children from eight schools, *rdo* holds [50]. Among four *V* for math-precocious kindergarten and preschoolers, *mo* always holds and *mdo* holds for three *V* [51]. Among eight *V* for reading and four *V* for math, *mdo* and *rdo* always hold [52, 53]. Among elementary Grades 2 through 6, five *V*, *mdo* always holds [54]. Among SAT assessments, *mdo* holds for all eight *V* [12]. In Johns Hopkins University talent searches employing the SAT math scores, *mdo* holds for all 10 *V* [55, 56]. Among twins assessed at ages 7, 9, and 10 and for three different math skills and one reading test at each age, *mo* and *ro* hold for all 12 *V* [57]. Lakin was noted above [7]. She reported standardization data implying 28 *V* with results spanning 27 years, for ages 9 to 17, 26 of 28 *V* satisfy *mo*, and *mdo* could not be evaluated. Among four *V* summarizing Taiwanese children's math test performance, four satisfied *mo*, and three satisfied *mdo* [58]. In an Australian sample for children of fifth year schooling for math *mdo* holds, while for reading $s_b > s_g$ fails [59]. Cascella [60] reports two large sample *V* based on fifth and tenth grade Italian children, both satisfy *mdo*. A massive 2013 Italian math study involved

"…the entire population of Italian children in school years 2, 5, 6, 8 and 10, [61, p. 4]." Reporting implied all years satisfy mo except year 5 where $s_b = s_g$. mdo could not be evaluated. Two V for sixth grade Kenyan children, one V for private schools, the other for public schools, both satisfy mdo [62]. Maccoby and Jacklin [53, p. 90] report two V for Project Talent where mdo holds for both and one ACT test V where mo holds but mdo fails. They report two other studies for which mo fails.

In the preceding paragraph, there is reference to 88 math V. All but nine appear independent of one another, and all but five V satisfy mo or mdo. For reading, reference is made to 35 V. All but three V appear independent of one another, and all but three satisfy ro or rdo.

2.3 Early Twentieth Century U.S. Reading and Math Tests

The earliest empirical findings on achievement test score sex differences provide a useful backdrop for viewing contemporary hypotheses regarding sex differences in math and reading achievement testing. There are, however, difficulties in assessing this early literature. While V are desired, they are infrequently available with the elements of V being replaced by other easier to compute quantities. However, it was evident early on that boys and girls differed both in their math and in their reading achievement test distributions as Gray and Stone reported in their 1917 and 1908 doctoral dissertations, respectively [3, 4]. These differences largely hold independent of age or grade level or type of test. The main exception would seem to be that girls exceed boys in tests of elementary arithmetic.

Remarkably, the early investigators tested large sample sizes which they could not hope to fully analyze given the tools available to them. The earliest U.S. achievement testing appears to have been initiated by J. M. Rice, a New York City educated physician who ended his practice in 1888, then studied psychology at universities in Leipzig and Jena, before turning his interest to achievement testing. He constructed achievement tests for both spelling and math. He reported in 1897 results of testing 33,000 children on his spelling test [1]. He then turned to math achievement testing. Rice was said by Stone to have developed the earliest math achievement test in the U.S.A. [3, p. 95]. Rice constructed eight arithmetic word problems for each grade, fourth through eighth, then ultimately tested 5,903 children in 18 schools in seven cities [2]. Rice never addressed issues of sex differences in test performance.

Around 1900, only paper and pencil calculation of any desired quantities was likely possible; not until 1902 was a printing calculator with addition and subtraction operations introduced. Only decades later would four operation machines be available [63]. Graphs were done manually as well and of course so was test scoring and evaluation. One result was that only a portion of the data collected were numerically summarized in some fashion. Because the sample mean and sample standard deviation required algebraic calculations, they were often replaced by easier to compute approximations. Thorndike wrote a book addressing the problem [64]. A key quantity for Thorndike was the median, which requires essentially only ordering data and counting. The median could replace the mean, and the median formed the basis for other approximations. The Average Deviation or $AD = \sum_x |x - M|/n$, where x denotes a test score, n is sample size, and M denoted the mean, or the median if the mean was not available. AD approximated the standard deviation. The coefficient of variation, $s/\bar{x}$, the sample standard deviation divided by the sample mean, could be replaced by AD/M. For Pearson's r, two approximations were suggested which, in examples Thorndike provided, were much larger than r, sometimes by 20% [64, p. 31].

One silver lining of these early computational difficulties may have been the tendency to report tabulated raw frequency data, sometimes with little comment other than what could be gleaned by a visual glance. Constructing tables of score frequencies would seem far easier than computing summary quantities by hand.

Most early U.S. sex difference studies are summarized by Lincoln (1927) [65] in numerous tables. Table and page references in this section below are all to Lincoln, unless noted otherwise. Lincoln's book was his Harvard education doctorate, and according to him, it was the first attempt to gather together sex difference research findings on a myriad of variables. Two earlier reviews actually appeared [66, 67] which Lincoln does not reference. This is understandable, however, because the sources report no useful numerical data.

There is clear evidence of mdo holding in the early literature. While V are reported for some math results, no V appear to have been reported for early reading results for reasons just noted. Already noted were Stone's [3] efforts constructing two tests, he called fundamental and reasoning, intended to assess sixth grade children. Others used his tests more widely. Based on the analysis of data, he reports [3, p. 30–32], and as noted earlier, one test satisfies mo, and the other mdo. Stone's test data will be analyzed in Chap. 5.

In his 1916 University of Chicago dissertation, Gray produced a series of oral and silent reading tests which were widely used early on (versions of which are used today). He was probably the first one to report sex differences in reading achievement. He provides no useful data for analysis, but his Diagram XIII [4, p. 127] is reproduced here as Fig. 2.1. "The diagram shows that in all grades girls do better than boys in oral reading [4, p. 126]."

Gray's tests were the basis for providing likely the first large scale assessment of reading achievement, in the 1918 Survey of the St. Louis Public Schools [68, 69] a massive work of which a portion was devoted to reading, writing, arithmetic, and music assessments; only for the reading tests are there data on sex differences. The volumes were intended as supporting documents for a proposed school bond offering.

Both the oral and silent reading tests developed by Gray were based on short paragraphs each child read, during which a child's time in seconds to read each paragraph was recorded, along with several types of reading errors. An oral reading score depended on the seconds taken to read each of twelve paragraphs together with the number of errors made. For silent reading, the length of time required to

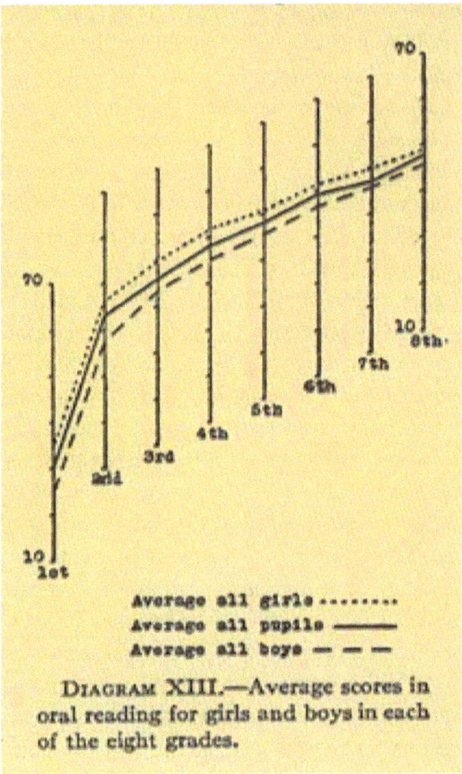

Fig. 2.1 Graph from Gray [4, p. 127] showing girls' mean exceeding boys' mean for Grades 1 to 8 on the Gray Oral reading test

read three short paragraphs determined a child's silent reading rate with answers provided to questions about the content read. The results are summarized in two tables in Lincoln which appeared earlier [69]. Table 35, based on 5,118 children, shows girls exceed boys in oral reading for Grades 1 to 8 at seven of eight grade levels. The silent reading test scores, Table 36, were based on 4,463 children with two performance indices, quality scores, and rate scores. For five grades, two through eight, boys exceed girls in all grades on quality, which presumably reflects the "...ability to master the thought of what is read [69, p. 170]." Using the reading rate score, or reading speed, girls exceed boys in four of the seven grade levels and are tied at one grade. The number of boys and girls at each grade in these tests was typically above 300.

Lincoln reports reading scores by other investigators and other tests in four additional tables. In all cases, the performance variable favors girls, sometimes by wide margins. Table 37 reports a before and after experiment comparing reading rates. For six grade levels at the beginning, girls' averages exceed boys' averages in five grades. At end, girls exceed boys in silent reading for four of six grades. Table 38 displays both rate and comprehension scores for six grades in rural Iowa. For both indices, girls exceed boys in five of six grade level comparisons. Table 39 reports quality scores at nine ages, 7 to 15; girls exceed boys in median scores at all ages.

And when speed was the performance variable, girls are vastly superior, at eight of nine ages, reported in Table 40. Concerning sex differences in reading variability, in three of four tables [65, pp. 149-154] with sex comparisons spanning ages 8 to 15 years, boys' reading test standard deviations exceed the standard deviation for girls in both quality and reading speed in five or more of seven comparisons in each table. Lincoln concludes "The weight of the evidence seems to indicate that girls are somewhat superior to boys in reading [65, p. 72]."

S. A. Courtis [70] constructed eight arithmetic tests of varying content that were used in a New York city school testing program around 1910. These tests will be considered in more detail later. Test 8, in Lincoln's Table 106, a reasoning test of eight word problems, was administered to 13,629 boys and 13,542 girls (probably in Grades 4 to 8); based on an analysis of these data and discussed further below, mdo holds. Brooks [71] used Stone's reasoning test. mo holds for 5 of 7 ages, 9 to 15. The results are in Table 34. Thorndike [72] constructed four arithmetic reasoning word problems. With substantial Massachusetts school personnel help, 4,640 children were tested. Reported were the percentage of boys exceeding the girls' median. In 22 of 24 comparisons, in an unnumbered table [65, p. 61] for grades 6 to 9, boys' percentage exceeded 50%, which might be a proxy for $\bar{x}_b > \bar{x}_g$. No index of variability is given. Interestingly, in a footnote, Lincoln reports that around 1917 Cyril Burt "...found the same difference in London schools [65, p. 60]." In yet an additional math reasoning test, spanning five grade levels, fourth through sixth, all 10 comparisons favored boys. The index was the percentage of boys exceeding the girls' median [65, p. 59].

From 1100 to 1200 New York city students of each sex were tested in each of 18 grade levels from forth to twelfth (e.g., 4A, 4B to 12A, 12B); results are given for two tests selected by Courtis which he thought revealed the greatest sex difference. Seventeen of the eighteen test medians, Table 27, favor girls on Test 3, a 120 item multiplication test of single-digit numbers (e.g., 3×4). Lincoln writes "There appears a very clear superiority in favor of girls [65, p. 57]." Turn the page for Table 28: for Courtis Test 6, a 16-item reasoning test, all word problems, Lincoln comments: "Here we find the differences largely in favor of boys... [65, p. 58];" 14 of 18 grades favored boys. These tables and associated commentary provide clear evidence, in large sample data, that early on it was recognized that girls exceeded boys on measures of central tendency for certain arithmetic tests.

In summary, the early literature does provide evidence of mdo and mo holding for arithmetic reasoning tests. It also demonstrates that very early in achievement testing's history, there was good evidence that girls exceed boys on certain arithmetic tests. Should V for reading have been reported, it appears that many studies would have satisfied ro and likely rdo as well.

As a historical note, it seems important to recognize E. L. Thorndike's impact on the early development of both math and reading achievement tests. From 1899 forward, Thorndike spent his entire career at Teacher's College, Columbia University. He was Stone's statistical and conceptual advisor on math achievement testing. Gray, a pioneer in reading tests, while earning his BA in 1913 and doctorate in 1916 from the University of Chicago, earned a master's at Columbia University in 1914, where he was influenced by Thorndike. Lincoln footnotes other Thorndike students, for example, Brooks [71]. For a very different perspective on Thorndike and his early influence, see Shields [73].

Chapter 3
Varying Viewpoints on Sex Differences

Conceptual deficiencies, the surprising claim of no math test score sex differences, and other efforts to understand or explain math and other sex differences in task performance are of concern here. Those readers primarily interested in methods, models, and subsequent results may skip to Chap. 4 with little loss in continuity.

3.1 Similarities and Hellinger Distances

When Hyde in 2005 introduced her similarities hypothesis which "...holds that males and females are similar on most but not all psychological variables [74, p. 581]," she could have given the idea of similarities, an old psychological concept, a rigorous definition, and at the same time, proposed another more appropriate index of sex differences. But this did not happen. d although widely used then as now, was well-recognized, at that time, to be a conceptually inadequate index of sex differences at least for some tasks. The need to report s_b^2/s_g^2 in addition to d clearly implies that recognition, at least implicitly. If the population variances of the two sexes were plausibly regarded as the same, there would be no need to report variance ratios. Furthermore, much earlier Feingold in 1992 [28] presciently argued, as noted earlier, that to understand sex differences, both means and variances must be addressed. Feingold seemed to be calling for a new conceptual model for sex differences. Just how this goal could be achieved was apparently not obvious, as there appears to have been no proposal to do so in the subsequent decades.

However, simply exchanging d and its model δ for an index that relaxes the population variance equality constraint would have been an important conceptual improvement. It might also have changed the psychology of how sex differences are viewed, away from the simple and misleading notion that sex differences are primarily, if not just exclusively, mean differences.

H. Thomas, *Sex Differences in Reading and Math Test Scores of Children*,
Monographs in the Psychology of Education,
https://doi.org/10.1007/978-3-031-41272-1_3

Instead, the notion of similarities and effect size d were tightly tied. In addition, there was no indication of just what variable attributes the similarities hypothesis were intended to capture other than effect size differences. Yet in the language of psychology, the notion of "psychological variable similarities" certainly extends well beyond the narrow effect size mean differences index [75]. The similarities hypothesis seems to have remained conceptually untethered to anything other than effect size and those often observed small values of $|d|$ in various tasks.

A more appropriate scalar index of sex differences that is easy to compute, assuming the variables of both sexes follow normality, is the Hellinger distance denoted as H [76]. H overcomes obvious deficiencies of d and unlike δ, H is a metric, that is, H is a measure of distance between a pair of probability distributions. It does require that the distributions of concern be specified, which is not required for δ. But distributional normality is implicitly assumed seemingly always, in settings where d is of focus, so this added assumption seems benign. H does not require equal population variance for both sexes, an Achilles heal for δ and consequently d. Under δ and thus d, two distributions are conceptualized as different by location-shift, obviously conceptually wrong at least for sex differences in reading and math test score distributions. H does not depend on how the distributions of boys and girls test scores are conceptualized as different. H is bounded in the interval zero to one, with zero indicating the distributions are identical and one if the distributions are disjoint.

H and a function of H for use in what follows will be defined below in Chap. 4. As a scalar, estimates of H make it easy to compare the differences, in for example, boys' and girls' PISA math test score distributions for different countries, assuming V are available. Thus H can put the issue of U.S. test score sex differences into a broader global perspective. H could provide a unifying common sex differences metric that reflects variance differences even if variances were otherwise ignored. Any alternative index proposed is unlikely to replace d because d is too well ingrained in the fabric of research. But perhaps H can be reported along with d. H has a clear conceptual interpretation as a distance. d has no clear interpretation, at least for sex differences in reading and math test scores.

One might observe that what Hyde seemed to have wanted, with her similarities hypothesis, was a *metric* or distance index on the separation of probability distributions of boys and girls on whatever the current variable of interest happened to be. She writes "Crucial to meta-analysis is the concept of effect size, which measures the *magnitude* of an effect—in this case the *magnitude* of gender difference [74, p. 582, italics added]." The word "magnitude," which Hyde used repeatedly, usually carries with it in science at least the notion of a distance or metric, a property that the index she was advocating lacked. To write "measures the magnitude" clearly suggests Hyde wanted a "yard stick" which she did not have.

3.2 The False Claim of Parity in Math Testing

In 2019, Hyde and others [15] cite a large-scale meta-analysis [9] and conclude "...girls had reached parity with boys in mathematics [15, p. 177]." They report a second meta-analysis [10] which "... accumulated data from 242 studies, representing the testing of more than 1.2 million people. Overall, $d = 0.05$, again indicating no gender difference [15, p. 177]."

While these statements sound impressive and may seem initially compelling, sex differences in math achievement test score distributions have been recognized and well documented for more than 100 years [3, 70, 71]. Furthermore, data demonstrating these differences have long been available, as detailed in Chap. 2. Consequently, the claim that there are no gender differences in math test scores seems preposterous.

However, statements that boys and girls are "equal" in math performance [25, p. 377] show "no gender difference," the differences are "trivial or nonexistent," or that "parity" has been achieved [15, p. 177] or similar characterizations have appeared in publications spanning well more than a decade [9, 10, 15, 25, 32, 33]. Consequently, it is interesting to understand the basis for this remarkable "no gender difference" or "parity" in math testing claim, made by varying subsets of a set of 13 different researchers authoring the just referenced publications.

First, consider what a "no difference" claim actually means. The precise intended meaning of the claim seems unclear because it appears to have has never been explicitly defined. However, their argument rests on average d values from large-scale meta-analyses. Thus the claim is properly seen as a *conditional* claim because d addresses only mean differences in distributions, ignoring variance differences. But no conditions are placed on their summary statements. For example, "Our analysis shows that, for grades 2 to 11, the general population no longer shows a gender difference in math skills, consistent with the gender similarities hypothesis [9, p. 495]." This statement makes clear their claim is unconditional.

The only plausible approach to understanding is that the "parity" or "no gender differences" claims are to be taken as *equivalent* to the hypothesis that boys and girls share the same math achievement test score distributions. With this equivalency, the claims are easily dispatched without statistical concerns, using data they conveniently provide. Under the identical distribution hypothesis, as already noted, s_b^2/s_g^2, over studies, should fluctuate about one, while d should, over studies, fluctuate about zero. As discussed earlier in Chap. 1 in Table S1 [31] are listed 66 variance ratios; 65 are greater than one. Under the parity hypothesis, 33 would be expected to be so. In Table 7 [10, p. 1132] which reports NAEP data (and is similar to Table 2.1 here) are listed 36 variance ratios, all of which are greater than one; only 18 would be expected. In the same table are listed 36 d values; 34 are positive. Only 18 positive would be expected.

There is no surprise that this analysis shows the no difference hypothesis is false. While below their Table 7, the authors do state that "Overall, we conclude that a small gender difference favoring boys in complex problem solving is still present in high school [10, p. 1132]." That is not the message the authors wish to convey. In their abstract, they state "Overall, $d = 0.05$ indicating no gender difference ... [10, p. 1132]."

The puzzle is how these authors justify a no sex differences in math test scores claim when they must be aware of where such an elementary and obvious analysis leads. The answer appears easily given. The first and most important fact is that they ignore data consistencies in their reasoning. The foremost feature of data to recognize in addressing psychology's crisis, according to Kagan [34], is patterns in the data. The remarkably consistent outcome patterns of $d > 0$ and $s_b^2/s_g^2 > 1$ are clearly the most striking feature of their Table 7 [10, p. 1132] and immediately noticeable by anyone. Furthermore, this consistency is arguably the most striking feature of their article. This being so, it apparently does not matter how many small positive d there are or how many variance ratios greater than one there are, apparently for some readers and some of these authors, the no difference or parity claim is unshakeable.

The second fact is that often no standard errors or other indices of uncertainty are given for their summary quantities, typically values of $\bar{d}$. They simply report the statistic of interest and assert their belief. It needs to be acknowledged, however, that the construction of standard errors for meta-analysis may not be as straightforward as commonly believed. What are claimed as appropriate standard errors are often wrongly constructed. Shuster's research on these matters is convincing [77].

Set aside the state test data-based claim that "The weighted mean is 0.0065, consistent with no gender difference [9, p. 495];[31, p. 8]." The fact that 65 of 66 s_b^2/s_g^2 exceed one, in huge sample sizes, decisively falsifies any parity claim for these state math test data. This outcome consistency seems remarkable when it is recognized that how the different tests differ in math content is unknown, that the grade levels ranged from grade 2 to 11, and that likely there were wide ranges of differences in test administration, scoring, and recording procedures employed among the different states. Such consistency simply rarely occurs in the psychological literature. But given the fact that *mdo* widely holds, it is perhaps not surprising that a rejection of the parity idea for the state test data comes from variances, not means. It seems reasonable to suspect that the near-zero weighted $\bar{d}$ is because of the likely variability of the content of the state tests, keeping in mind that boys' advantage on math tests seems related to a test's reasoning component.

Similar subjectively judged decisions appear elsewhere. Referring to an earlier posting of NAEP data, similar to Table 2.3, Hyde writes "For these items, at grade 12, the average effect size was $d = 0.07$, indicating that girls had reached parity with boys even for complex problem solving at the high school level [25, p. 381]." And earlier in the same source appears "... girls' math performance is equal to that of boys... [25, p. 377]." Hyde reminds the reader she defined $d \leq 0.10$ as trivial [25, p. 379].

It is interesting to note that for the 31 math V, in Tables 2.1 and 2.3, all but one d are, by Hyde's definition, trivial. What is one expected to conclude? The answer apparently desired is that the remarkably consistent sex differences in the NAEP data gathered over decades, revealing small mean differences favoring boys, and at three grade levels, using the most sophisticated protocol in U.S. history, and involving millions of children, are to be dismissed as substantively trivial.

In summary, U.S. large sample representative data concerning sex differences in math testing show that for math tests with a reasoning component, the mean for boys is nearly always modestly larger than the mean for girls, and the variances for boys are nearly always far larger than the variance for girls. There appears no evidence this conclusion is inappropriate for nearly all international settings as well, at least for developed countries, as Table 2.5 reveals.

3.3 Sex Differences and Searching for Answers

Other researchers clearly recognize there exist, and have existed, sex differences in math testing, as well as reading. A key question is why such differences occur. Efforts to find definitive answers in test score data have largely failed. The most recent efforts have focused on math testing. As an example, Italian children's PISA math gap, which is the mean sex difference favoring boys, has been among the largest in Europe. To understand why, the 2013 Italian national assessment examination, the INVALSI, for school years 2, 5, 6, 8, and 10 was examined [61]. The "sample" was the entire population of school children's scores, more than 125,859 tests. Employing what they term as dynamic regression models, the effort yielded no definitive answers, but they conclude "... girls systematically underperform boys, even after controlling for an array of individual and family background characteristics, and that the average gap increases with children's age [61, p. 1]." In a rewrite, they suggest stereotypes play a major role in both reading and math test score sex differences. Although understanding the PISA math mean sex difference was the motivation for their study, they write in closing: "The analysis of the reasons why the gender gap in math exists and how it can be reduced is beyond the scope of our contribution [78, p. 39]."

Stereotypes regarding girls and women have long been viewed as important variables for degrading girls' and women's test performance and thus explaining sex differences in math performance, as the previous [78] study illustrates. This perspective is a recurring theme in the math sex differences literature [79]. Stereotype threat has been well researched and has been shown, in some studies, to deleteriously impact on girls' math test scores [80]. Boys' reading scores can be similarly influenced [81]. However, after assessing 15 years of evidence, it was concluded stereotype threat is unlikely to importantly influence girls' math performance [82]. Even if the results had turned out differently and stereotype threat were shown to be a viable and important variable, because variance differences were ignored, the results would be unable to address the core concern here: how the inequalities noted at the outset, in $\mathcal{S}$, originate and why do they persist.

Six variables are said to mediate sex differences in math [83]: 1-Stereotype threat, 2-ostracism and gender identification, 3-self-sufficiency, 4-teacher and parent factors, 5-math-related experiences, and 6-math test anxiety. Evidence is cited for each. Collectively, it is argued "It has simply never been established that there is any meaningful and substantial sex difference in mathematics ability that is not massively confounded with factors related to individual experience [83, p. 42]." If true, these facts would seem to only magnify the importance of understanding the inequalities of focus here because they have managed to "poke through" the massive confounding claimed and nearly universally appear in the summary sample statistics. It is difficult, however, to see the relevance of such research on sex differences of primary concern here. That is because, again, of the failure to consider what are, after all, the largest sex differences, the variance differences.

A multiyear Herculean effort reviewing more than four hundred publications culminated in Ceci, Williams, and Barnett [84, 85] and a corresponding lower-key book [5]. Their explicit, well-defined, and important main target goal was to explain the observed frequency participation differences among men and women in scientific and math-related occupations. This is not an explicit concern addressed here, but many issues they address overlap with issues of focus here. Yet at the end, it was not possible to find any explicit statement rendered by these authors regarding why such frequency differences between the sexes exist, and persist, and at different rates in different countries often with differences in languages and in different cultures.

There is a literature, to be noted below, which specifically addresses similar frequency differences in success rates observed in boys' and girls' performances on certain cognitive tasks. Such findings, if they had been considered, could have been suggestive of corresponding sex differences in adults. Consequently, a different conclusion might have been provided than the one expressed: "...we believe that the evidence...points to nonbiological/ability factors as the *major* causes of the underrepresentation of women in mathematically intensive careers [5, p. xii; italics in original]."

The strategy here, as noted earlier, is to explicitly focus on the specific set of empirical conditions of $\mathcal{S}$, as the target for theoretical explanation. This narrow strategy may ultimately lead to greater overall understanding of sex differences than framing a far larger more encompassing set of goals.

3.4 Genetics: The Oldest Recognized Sex Differences Influence

Genetical X-linked influences have been recognized since the Talmud [86]. Furthermore, their trait influence is thought to be stable, with change occurring very slowly over long periods of time [87]. It is notable that interest in sex differences has probably always been triggered by frequency disparities in task performance, often most easily recognized in observational settings.

O'Connor in 1943 [88] appears to have been the first to propose that X-linked gene influences could explain behavioral sex differences in performance unexplainable within alternative frameworks. Boys outperformed girls on his "wiggly blocks" task. In brief, given an X-linked gene in two alleles, if the recessive form has relative frequency q and is performance enhancing, then the proportion of q boys should exceed the proportion of q^2 girls. Or alternatively, the mean task performance for the boys should exceed the mean task performance for girls.

However, not until the 1960 to 1980 interval were there efforts to address O'Connor's suggestion. The earliest approaches involved familial correlations. While a correlational approach cannot address the inequalities of focus here, this early history appears to have continued to shape perspectives today and in unhelpful ways.

Under a bivariate discrete binary outcome X-linked Mendelian model (each marginal distribution is Bernoulli, with 0 or 1 outcome), the expected correlations among pairs of related individuals, for example, mother-daughter, or sister-brother, can be specified, given only the gene frequency. However, measurements on variables possibly mediated by X-linked influences are typically observations on outcome variables such as achievement test scores typically regarded as continuously distributed. It was widely assumed, wrongly, that continuous bivariate test score correlations could serve as a proxy for estimating the desired discrete Mendelian correlations. The general failure of the correlations computed on continuous data to yield what was hoped to be estimates of the Mendelian correlations, provoked strong rebukes concerning even the possibility of X-linked effects. For example, "the validity of the hypothesis is unfounded [89]," or "Sex differences... Not an X-linked effect [90]."

What went unrecognized was a conceptual problem: there was no basis for assuming a discrete bivariate Mendelian correlation could be estimated from correlations obtained from continuous bivariate test score model. Indeed, it was shown that attempting to construct a conceptual basis for doing so was essentially analytically impossible or at least intractable [91].

The consequence of this result implied these early correlational approaches were misguided and conceptually flawed. Nevertheless, the general failure of a correlation approach, along with the strongly worded, largely condemnatory spirit of the attacks appears to have carried over to present times. Indeed, the very idea that one might believe any trait might be attributable to a single-gene effect signals to some writers, even today, that such persons are beyond redemption and also are apparently stupid: "An education in psychology is not sufficient to overcome the appeal of single genes [92, p. 495]." It may well be these authors wish to reconsider their belief. A *single gene* TKTL1 may well be responsible for distinguishing cognitive abilities of modern humans from Neanderthals [93].

Besides the fact that genetical arguments are often, understandably, psychologically unappealing, there was another issue. Many X-linked recessive traits are deleterious, and some lethal, and suggesting a recessive gene might enhance performance seemed implausible, especially given the role of dominance in the theory of natural selection [94, 95]. This perspective has been revised, and today the role of recessive genes as having beneficial effects is an active area of research [96].

The acknowledgment of X-linkage as a possible factor explaining sex differences remains largely absent in the contemporary psychological sex differences literature concerning reading and math, although not the wider literature addressing sex differences more generally. The possibility of other forms of genetical influence, namely polygene effects playing a role in observed sex differences, seems more widely acknowledged, in the psychological literature, although rarely explicitly embraced, at least in the recent psychological sex differences literature.

An important notable earlier exception to this recent trend are the perspectives of Eleanor Maccoby and Carol Jacklin [53]. In their time, they were arguably the most scholarly, the most influential, authoritative, and unbiased voices on matters of sex differences. They argued, far more broadly than is being argued here, that the origins of psychological sex differences were determined by "...certain sex-linked biological predispositions, but to say so is not to deny the importance of social learning. [53, p. 275]." Their entire book is framed within a biological perspective. Consider their book-ending section title: "Is Biology Destiny? [53, p. 373]." They clearly embraced the likelihood of biological factors playing a role by setting boundary conditions: "A variety of social institutions are viable within the framework set by biology [53, p. 374]." And they addressed explicitly, and in some detail, the possibility of recessive X-linkage as a possible sex differences factor in spatial task settings [53, pp. 121–122; 361].

Part of the reluctance to embrace genetical influences is understandable: one reason is there is often missing any explicit convincing mechanistic connection between general statements of genetical influences on sex differences, and the observed sex differences that triggered the interest in the first place, such as the observed relative frequency differences arising on certain task performances, or the obvious lopsided participation rates among men and women in certain math-oriented occupations. A coherent conceptual framework is needed which accounts for these observational differences and which also accounts for the summary statistical inequalities.

If math talent is facilitated by an X-linked recessive gene, all sons of math talented women, twelve Israeli university mathematicians, should be math talented. Math talent was defined as an SAT math score greater than 700. Among ten women who agreed to participate, all six boys were talented. Of ten girls, one was expected to be talented, but none were. Hypothesizing that each sex is equally likely to be talented is easily rejected $p < 0.0004$. While small, the study [97] is remarkable.

With varying methodological approaches, X-linked explanations have accounted for observed sex differences in Piaget's water-level task [98, 99], the mental rotation task [100], variance differences in intelligence [101], but see [102]; in addition, there have been explanations for sex differences in performance on Witkin's rod and frame task [103] and gifted students' math test performance [104].

More recently, there has been a wide recognition of the plausibility that X-linked genetical factors can contribute to phenotypical behavioral differences between boys and girls [87, 105–108]. In addition, the documented importance of X-linkage for understanding trait distribution continues to grow [109].

Chapter 4
Genetical and $\mathcal{Y}$ Models for Math and Reading

This chapter details first the genetical model and then the probability model $\mathcal{Y}$ for math and reading. While the formality of the approach is distinctive, crucial to the endeavor is just how sex differences are construed. Rather than to focus on *between* sex differences, the focus is on *within* sex differences. This is the key to conceptual understanding.

It is this focus on within sex differences, not between sex differences, which appears to set the approach apart from all other efforts to explain sex differences. Viewing matters from an effect size perspective is simply putting on a conceptual blindfold. Once these within sex differences are suitably modeled, the framework for understanding the between sex differences follows nearly trivially.

Only the model specifications and results of the analyses appear below. The arguments appear in Appendix A. The most important analytical results state that the inequality orderings on the parameters of $\mathcal{Y}$ correspond with the empirical inequalities of mo and mdo in the case of math and ro and rdo in the case of reading. Consequently, the elements of $\mathcal{S}$ are simply *expectations* under $\mathcal{Y}$.

Two "toy" examples to hopefully aid intuition and illustrate the model's usefulness in both generating data and estimating parameters appear at the start of Chap. 5. The moment estimation procedure is detailed in Appendix A.3, and an R code implementation [110] is given in Appendix A.4.

4.1 The Genetical Model

"X-linked genes, especially escape genes... contribute to sex differences [105, p. 241]." X-linkage, also referred to as sex-linkage, is applied here to math and reading test score sex differences in boys and girls. Recall boys have X and Y chromosomes, Y inherited from their father and X from their mother. Girls have two X chromosomes, one from their father and one from their mother. For girls,

H. Thomas, *Sex Differences in Reading and Math Test Scores of Children*, Monographs in the Psychology of Education,
https://doi.org/10.1007/978-3-031-41272-1_4

the genes of one of these X chromosomes are mostly inactivated, but some genes escape this inactivation. Considering biallelic genes that escape inactivation, girls have genotypes AA, Aa, aA, and aa, while boys with a single X have genotypes A or a, with capital A denoting the dominant and lower case a the recessive allele. Assume for girls AA, Aa, and aA all lead to the same phenotypic test performance for girls as does A for boys. Assume a boys and aa girls display identical test score performance. Assume A and a have relative frequencies $\Pr(A) = p \in (0, 1)$, $\Pr(a) = q \in (0, 1)$, and $p + q = 1$. Assume girls' four genotypes AA, aA, Aa, and aa follow a binomial with $(p+q)^2 = p^2 + 2pq + q^2$ with $\Pr(aa) = q^2$. The pairs of probabilities of focus: for girls q^2 and $1 - q^2$ and for boys q and $1 - q$.

In math, a and aa with probabilities q and q^2, respectively, for boys and girls, are assumed to facilitate high math performance. They become coefficients of latent probability distributions in the probability model to explain sex differences in high math test score performance. For reading, a gene with allele frequencies $1 - q$ and $1 - q^2$ is assumed to facilitate high reading performance for boys and girls, respectively, and these too become coefficients of latent reading distributions. Of course, different genes are assumed to be involved for each task.

4.2 Model $\mathcal{Y}$ for Math

The fundamental idea is that there are, for boys' and girls' math and reading test scores, two latent unobserved subpopulations within each sex. The shapes of these two subpopulations define the shape of each sex's population, that is, each sex's test score distribution. One subpopulation is composed of high scoring individuals, and the other subpopulation is composed of low scoring individuals. It is assumed all individuals are members of one, and only one, of these subpopulations. Assume for the moment that all high scoring individuals, both boys and girls, have outcomes μ_2, while all low scoring individuals have outcome μ_1 with $\mu_1 < \mu_2$. μ_1 and μ_2 are outcomes of a binary two-outcome "Bernoulli-like" random variable B: B_b for boys and B_g for girls. While B_b and B_g have identical outcomes, their outcome probabilities are different.

Now focus on math. The probability of $B_b = \mu_2$ is q or $P(B_b = \mu_2) = q$ and $P(B_b = \mu_1) = 1 - q$. For girls, $P(B_g = \mu_2) = q^2$ and $P(B_g = \mu_1) = 1 - q^2$. So the probability of the B outcomes reflects the gene frequencies just given above, with the recessive gene facilitating higher test scores for math.

Of course, the outcomes of test scores are not discrete binary outcomes μ_1 or μ_2. Rather they are usually regarded as continuous. Thus, another random variable is required, N: it is assumed to be independent of B, and it has mean zero and variance $\sigma^2 > 0$, and like B_b and B_g, there is a pair, N_b for boys and N_g for girls. N_b and N_g have identical but unspecified distributions and reflect other sources of variance influencing test scores.

So far, all the above theory is latent and unobserved. What is observed is the additive composition of N and B. The result of this addition is that μ_1 and μ_2 become the means of two latent probability distributions which represent the two subpopulations.

Define $\mathcal{Y}$ by $Y = B + N$ where a realization of Y, that is, y, is a math test score and where

$$Y = B + N = \begin{cases} Y_b = B_b + N_b & \text{math for boys,} \\ Y_g = B_g + N_g & \text{math for girls.} \end{cases} \tag{4.1}$$

With E(·) denoting expectation and var(·) denoting variance,

$\mathrm{E}(Y_b) = \mu_b = (1-q)\mu_1 + q\mu_2$ and $\mathrm{E}(Y_g) = \mu_g = (1-q^2)\mu_1 + q^2\mu_2$.
$\mathrm{var}(Y_b) = \sigma_b^2 = q(1-q)(\mu_2-\mu_1)^2 + \sigma^2$; $\mathrm{var}(Y_g) = \sigma_g^2 = q^2(1-q^2)(\mu_2 - \mu_1)^2 + \sigma^2$.

Only realizations of Y_b and Y_g are observed. Importantly, the *only* sex differences are the discrete outcome probabilities for B_b and B_g given above. The distributions of Y_b and Y_g, along with three inequalities, may be given.

The Y_b and Y_g distributions are

$$f_b(y) = (1-q)f_1(y) + qf_2(y) \text{ the distribution for boys}$$

and

$$f_g(y) = (1-q^2)f_1(y) + q^2 f_2(y) \text{ the distribution for girls.}$$

$f_k(y) = f(y; \mu_k, \sigma^2), k = 1, 2$, and f is the distribution of N_b and N_g; f can be either continuous or discrete and is otherwise unspecified. Please see Appendix A.1 for the argument.

The distribution of Y_b is not the same as the distribution of Y_g plus a constant, provided $0 < q < 1$. Thus, $\mathcal{Y}$ is not a location-shift model. The right sides of $f_b(y)$ and $f_g(y)$ are latent and unobserved. But their parameters q, μ_1, μ_2, and σ^2 can be estimated, as will be illustrated in the next chapter.

The corresponding lower tail distribution functions $F_b(y)$ for boys and $F_g(y)$ for girls are (if y is continuous)

$$F_b(y) = (1-q)\int_{-\infty}^{y} f_1(w)dw + q\int_{-\infty}^{y} f_2(w)dw.$$

$$F_g(y) = (1-q^2)\int_{-\infty}^{y} f_1(w)dw + q^2\int_{-\infty}^{y} f_2(w)dw.$$

Again, $f_k(y) = f(y; \mu_k, \sigma^2), k = 1, 2$, and f is the distribution of N_b and N_g.

The population analogs of the empirical inequalities *mo* and *mdo* are given in the following three inequalities:

$$\mathrm{E}(Y_b) = \mu_b > \mu_g = \mathrm{E}(Y_g) \tag{4.2}$$

$$\mathrm{var}(Y_b) = \sigma_b^2 > \sigma_g^2 = \mathrm{var}(Y_g) \text{ and } \sigma_b > \sigma_g \text{ if } 0 < q < .618 \tag{4.3}$$

$$\sigma_b^2 - \sigma_g^2 > \mu_b - \mu_g \text{ given that (4.2), (4.3) and } L \text{ hold.} \tag{4.4}$$

$L = \{\mu_d = \mu_2 - \mu_1 > 1 \;\&\; 0 < q < ([5 - 4/\mu_d]^{1/2} - 1)/2 < .618\}$. L is a weak condition, requiring only that $\mu_2 - \mu_1 > 1$ and like (4.3) fixes an upper bound on the size of q. Please see Appendix A.2 for the arguments.

Inequalities (4.2), (4.3), and (4.4) reveal $\mathcal{Y}$ is easily falsifiable. In (4.4) that (4.2), (4.3) and L hold. Thus, failures in data of *mo* or *mdo* to hold might be taken as falsifying $\mathcal{Y}$, although sampling variability must be considered. Clearly, by inspection, $\mathrm{E}(Y_b)$ and $\mathrm{var}(Y_b)$ share common parameters and are functionally related and similarly for girls.

The key point in the above development is that $\mathcal{Y}$ generates the same analytical inequality orderings, in the model, inequalities (4.2), (4.3), and (4.4), as are observed in data, namely *mo* and *mdo*. Thus, under $\mathcal{Y}$, *mo* and *mdo* are expected outcomes.

4.3 Model $\mathcal{Y}$ for Reading

The reading model is analytically similar to the model for math. For math, the recessive gene is assumed to code for higher scores. For reading, the recessive gene with frequency q is assumed to be deleterious and thus codes for lower reading test scores. From a model perspective, the values of q and $1 - q$ for boys and q^2 and $1 - q^2$ for girls are interchanged wherever they appear: thus, q^2 is interchanged with $1 - q^2$ for girls, while $1 - q$ is interchanged with q for boys. Two inequalities change: $\mu_g > \mu_b$ and $\sigma_b^2 - \sigma_g^2 > \mu_g - \mu_b$. The distributions $f_b(y)$ and $f_g(y)$ for reading simply interchange their right-side coefficients of $f_k(y), k = 1, 2$. As with $\mathcal{Y}$ for math, the observed inequalities *ro* and *rdo* are simply expectations under $\mathcal{Y}$ for reading.

Different genes are assumed to underpin performance in math than underpin performance in reading. q is used to denote the gene frequencies in either case because, in almost all cases, no confusion should result in whether the q refers to reading or math. Occasionally, q may refer to either or both tasks. When confusion seems possible and the distinction is important, q_m and q_r, respectively, for math and reading q will distinguish the settings. Hats denote estimates for all parameters, e.g., $\hat{q}$ for the q estimate and $\hat{\sigma}$ for the σ estimate.

4.4 Hellinger Distance H

The Hellinger distance [76] will be used to measure the distance between the probability distributions of boys and girls in some illustrative examples in Chap. 5. H is a metric, that is, a distance, unlike δ the model for d. δ assumes equal population variances while H does not. For continuous data, the square of the distance between the boys' and girls' probability distributions is

$$H^2 = 1 - \int \sqrt{f_b(y) f_g(y)} dy.$$

H is zero if the two probability distributions are identical, and H is one if the two probability distributions do not share the same support; that is, their distributions over the horizontal axis are disjoint. For some continuous distributions, including the normal, there are algebraic expressions requiring only the parameters and which do not require integration [76].

Boys' and girls' test score distributions are usually quite similar and often are nearly identical. They share the same support, that is, boys and girls share the same test score outcomes. The result is that the estimated H values are often very small. Consequently, reported below are estimates of $Hd = 100H$. Hd remains a distance, scaled between zero and one hundred.

Chapter 5
Model Estimation and Illustration of Test Score Distributions

Parameter estimates under $\mathcal{Y}$ are provided for several reading and math test V and their estimated test score distributions from a variety of settings around the world, along with their graphic portrayals.

While model estimates can be provided for nearly all V which satisfy mo or ro, the only samples to be considered below are those that appear to be representative of the larger population. V for SAT tests, although as noted in Chap. 2 well satisfy mdo, will not be considered. That is because people who take the SAT choose to do so, and so they certainly do not reflect a more general population.

All data explored below are either contained herein or are easily accessible online. As noted earlier, the estimation algorithm is given in Appendix A.3, while an R code implementation [110] appears in Appendix A.4. Those V chosen as examples below illustrate similarities and contrasts for difference settings.

5.1 Math Examples

To assist understanding of $\mathcal{Y}$, defined as Equation 4.1 and discussed in Chap. 4, are two toy examples. Both masquerade as math test score settings. And both illustrate the ease of generating data under $\mathcal{Y}$ and the corresponding estimation of parameters. Implementation using coins and poker chips can cause some tedium.

5.1.1 Example 1: Coin Tosses

On one side of each of two pennies, mark 0, and on the other side, mark 10. On one side of a nickel, mark 5, and on the other side, mark −5. To simulate a virtual boy's test score, flip one penny and the nickel. The penny plays the role of the

H. Thomas, *Sex Differences in Reading and Math Test Scores of Children*, Monographs in the Psychology of Education,
https://doi.org/10.1007/978-3-031-41272-1_5

random variable B_b with outcomes 0 and 10, each with probability $q = 1/2$. The nickel plays the role of the random variable N_b with outcomes -5 and 5, each with probability one-half. Record the sum of the observed outcomes of both coins. This sum is a realized value y of Y_b from the model $Y_b = B_b + N_b$. Now repeat 100 times, thus obtaining "test scores" for 100 virtual boys.

Perhaps the following may further aid intuition: suppose the penny tossed for boys lands 0. Then following the nickel's toss, the outcome of the summed values is either -5 or 5. Should the penny have landed 10, the corresponding summed outcome following the nickel's toss would be 5 or 15. Thus, the two penny outcomes, 0 or 10, are each the centers of two distributions each with variance 25, the nickel's variance, resulting in a two-component mixture distribution with component means 0 and 10 and component variance 25. Each component's weight coefficient is one-half the penny's outcome probabilities. This paragraph completely specifies a discrete two-component mixture distribution.

For girls, flip all three coins. If both pennies show 10, take the value shown on the nickel, add 10, and record. If the outcome for the pennies is otherwise, simply record the outcome shown on the nickel. The two pennies play the role of B_g with outcome 10 with probability $q^2 = 1/4$ and zero with probability $1 - q^2 = 3/4$. The nickel plays for girls the role of N_g. The result is a realized value y of $Y_g = B_g + N_g$. Repeat the procedure 100 times, recording the data for 100 virtual girls. The possible outcomes for both sexes are $-5, 5$, and 15. One V realization is

$$V = \{\bar{x}_b = 5, \bar{x}_g = 2.400, s_b = 7.247, s_g = 6.454, n_b = 100, n_g = 100\},$$

which satisfies mdo. Below are the estimates, with hats, and the parameter values in parentheses:

$$\begin{aligned}
&\hat{q} = 0.396(q = 0.5),\\
&\hat{q}^2 = 0.157(q^2 = 0.25),\\
&\hat{\mu}_1 = 0.694(\mu_1 = 0),\\
&\hat{\mu}_2 = 11.562(\mu_2 = 10), \text{ and}\\
&\hat{\sigma}^2 = 25.142(\sigma^2 = 25).
\end{aligned}$$

5.1.2 Example 2: Poker Chips in Three Urns

Three urns are labeled B_b and B_g the boys' urn and girls' urn, respectively, and N. B_b contains 40 chips labeled 4 and 60 labeled 2; B_g contains 16 chips labeled 4 and 84 chips labeled 2. N contains 50 chips labeled -2 and 50 labeled 2. For boys sample with replacement, one chip from urn B_b and one from urn N (which may be thought of as a value of N_b) add the numbers, save the result, and repeat 100 times. Repeat the process for girls except urn B_g is used. Thus, there are 100 virtual "observations" for each sex. The possible outcomes are 0, 2, 4, and 6. A V

realization is

$$V = \{\bar{x}_b = 2.780, \bar{x}_g = 1.980, s_b = 2.272, s_g = 1.980, n_b = 100, n_g = 100\}.$$

The elements of V satisfy mdo. The parameter estimates have hats with parameter values in parentheses:

$$\begin{aligned}
&\hat{q} = 0.355(q = 0.400),\\
&\hat{q}^2 = 0.126(q^2 = 0.160),\\
&\hat{\mu}_1 = 1.540, (\mu_1 = 2),\\
&\hat{\mu}_2 = 5.033(\mu_2 = 4) \text{ and}\\
&\hat{\sigma}^2 = 2.471(\sigma^2 = 4).
\end{aligned}$$

$\mathcal{Y}$ for each sex is a mixture model with two latent component distributions $f_1(y)$ and $f_2(y)$. The two most important decisions usually encountered in constructing mixture models are first, the specification of the number of components. Here there are always two for each sex. The second concern is the specification of the latent unobserved component distributions. In most mixture models, the latent components are assumed to be normal distributions. However, typically there is no theory or empirical basis for justifying their specification. A wrong specification of the component distributions can lead to misunderstandings and inappropriate conclusions. There is usually no easy way to assess the consequences of wrongly specifying the mixture components, and thus criticisms or concerns that the components might be wrongly specified are difficult to counter. This problem is perhaps the central concern of many critics of the latent variables mixture model approach to understanding individual differences.

This concern is not relevant here because under $\mathcal{Y}$, as noted earlier, $f_1(y)$ and $f_2(y)$ the component distributions do not require specification for their parameters to be estimated. They can be any probability distribution, discrete or continuous. Consequently, $\mathcal{Y}$ consists of a pair of weak semiparametric mixture models. However, to construct graphs of the corresponding solutions provided below, the components must be specified. Thus *post* estimation, when component distributions graphically appear, they are constructed assuming the component distributions $f_1(y)$ and $f_2(y)$ are normal distributions.

An additional unusual advantage of the current estimation procedure, very unlike most solutions of finite mixtures, is that the solutions are closed form. That is, the solution output will always be the same with the same V input. In conventional mixture solutions, unlike the special situation here, and where the components are assumed to be normal distributions, iterative procedures often with randomly specified starting conditions are required. Consequently, the same mixture solution, given identical inputs with each solution, cannot be guaranteed.

5.1.3 Example 3: Italian Math Test

Considerably, more detail will accompany this example which may serve as a guide for interpreting the remaining examples for both math and reading. Cascella in 2020 [60] reported the large sample testing of Italian children, Grades 5 and 10, using the Italian INVALSI math achievement test. For both grades, *mdo* is satisfied. Grade 5 children, aged 10 years, are considered here.

The starting point is the summary statistics data vector V the only information. $V = \{\bar{x}_b = 198.913, \bar{x}_g = 191.881, s_b = 43.058, s_g = 39.845, n_b = 15453, n_g = 15415\}$.

$$\widehat{V} = \{198.913, 191.985, 43.065, 39.837\}.$$

$\widehat{V}$ is given here for easy comparison with V and will be explained momentarily below. Below are the parameter estimates with standard errors in parentheses:

$$\begin{aligned}
\hat{q} &= 0.178(0.023),\\
\hat{q}^2 &= 0.032(0.010),\\
\hat{\mu}_1 &= 190.362(0.572),\\
\hat{\mu}_2 &= 238.492(4.34), \text{ and}\\
\hat{\sigma}^2 &= 1516.197(21.59).
\end{aligned}$$

Define X-linked heritability for boys as

$$h_{bx}^2 = \widehat{\mathrm{var}}(B_b)/\widehat{\mathrm{var}}(Y_b)$$

and similarly for girls. $h_{bx}^2 = 0.182(0.015)$ and for girls $h_{gx}^2 = 0.045(0.007)$.

Once the parameter estimates are obtained, the predicted values are reported in $\widehat{V}$. These values may be compared with the observed values in V. The differences between V and $\widehat{V}$ may be taken as an index of how well the model accounts for the data. The elements of $\widehat{V}$ are the estimated values of the sample means and sample standard deviations, given the model estimates, and are computed from the parameter estimates where the estimates replace the model parameter values. Thus, these are approximately the expected values given the model estimates. The expressions to do so are given above in Chap. 4.

For example, the boys' predicted value of $\bar{y}$, which is 198.913 in this example, is the estimated expected value

$$\widehat{\mathrm{E}}(Y_b) = (1 - \hat{q})\hat{\mu}_1 + \hat{q}\hat{\mu}_2.$$

The girls' predicted standard deviation s_g is $\sqrt{\widehat{\mathrm{var}}(Y_g)}$ with

$$\widehat{\mathrm{var}}(Y_g) = (\hat{\mu}_2 - \hat{\mu}_1)^2\hat{q}^2(1 - \hat{q}^2) + \hat{\sigma}^2.$$

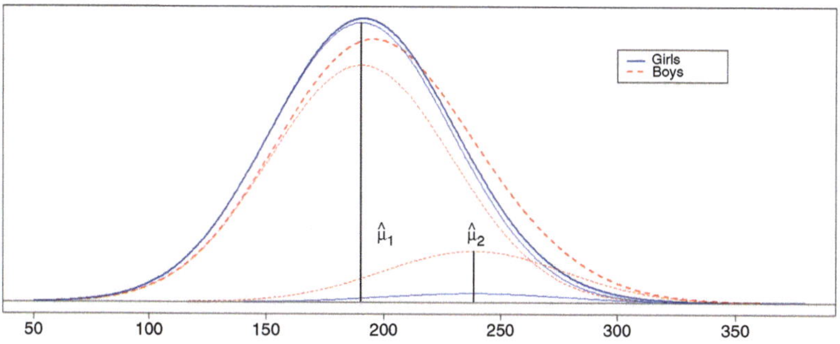

Fig. 5.1 Example 3. Thick lines are $\hat{f}_b(y)$ for boys and $\hat{f}_g(y)$ girls, and thin lines are their two components. The ordinates are at $\hat{\mu}_1$ and $\hat{\mu}_2$

In this example, it is 39.837. As the above comparison of V and $\widehat{V}$ reveals, the model estimates are in excellent agreement with the data.

Figure 5.1 provides a graphical solution with the post estimation assumption that $f_1(y)$ and $f_2(y)$, the latent components, are normally distributed. The estimated means of these two latent component distributions are shown by the vertical ordinates at the locations of $\hat{\mu}_1$ and $\hat{\mu}_2$, the estimated component means. The component distributions for both boys and girls share the same standard deviation, $\hat{\sigma} = 38.94$. The two bold lines, dashed and solid, are the estimates of $f_b(y)$ and $f_g(y)$, namely the estimated population models for boys and girls, respectively. If the test scores of the 30,868 children were available, these bold lines should resemble the histograms for boys and girls separately if the latent normal component distributions are reasonable specifications. The bold lines are determined by the thin lines of the unobserved components. There is a pair of thin lines for each sex. The two much smaller, thinner lines in the upper tails represent the distributions for boys (dashed lines) and girls (solid lines) for higher scoring latent component distributions. The shapes of these component distributions for boys and girls are identical; the girls' component is smaller because the weight $\hat{q}^2$ associated with this component is smaller for girls than the $\hat{q}$ weight for boys.

In particular, these two upper tail components with their estimated coefficient weights are $\hat{q}^2\hat{f}_2(y) = 0.032\hat{f}_2(y)$ for girls, and for boys it is $\hat{q}\hat{f}_2(y) = 0.178\hat{f}_2(y)$. $\hat{f}_1(y)$ and $\hat{f}_2(y)$ denote the probability distributions with estimates replacing their parameters. The other pair of thin lines, in the lower tails, are those associated with the boys' and girls' latent lower score component, $f_1(y)$. The girls' lower scoring component thin solid line is graphically indistinguishable in some regions of the graph. Precisely, these are $(1-\hat{q}^2)\hat{f}_1(y) = 0.968\hat{f}_1(y)$ for girls and $(1-\hat{q})\hat{f}_1(y) = 0.822\hat{f}_1(y)$ for boys. The girls' lower scoring weighted component line tracks the girls' $\hat{f}_g(y)$ closely because the lower component weight 0.968 is nearly one. The boys' lower scoring weighted component tracks $\hat{f}_b(y)$ less closely in most of the regions of the graph because the lower score component weight for the boys departs more sharply from one, namely 0.822.

The upper tail of $\hat{f}_b(y)$ for boys clearly shows more probability mass than the corresponding upper upper tail region of $\hat{f}_g(y)$ for the girls. It is commonly observed, e.g., [11], that upper tail region for boys' distribution "is fatter" than the distribution for girls. This figure, Fig. 5.1, illustrates that $\mathcal{Y}$ can explain this fact. An analytically based explanation will be provided later in Chap. 6.

In Fig. 5.1, the lines associated with the lower scoring weighted latent probability distributions, for both boys and girls, extend well above 250. Neither the model, $\mathcal{Y}$ nor the data imply, as mistakenly might be thought, that higher scoring boys or girls only come from the higher scoring component. While probabilities depend on the test score taken as the reference point (the lower limit of an integral), in fact, in this example, more higher scoring boys and girls can come from the lower than from the higher scoring components. To make this important point precise and using the equations defined in Chap. 4, the total estimated proportion of girls above $\hat{\mu}_2 \approx 238$ is $0.123 = 1 - \hat{F}_g(238)$, while $(1 - \hat{q}^2) \int_{238}^{\infty} \hat{f}_1(y)dy = 0.107$ the area under the girl's weighted lower scoring component but above 238 and $\hat{q}^2 \int_{238}^{\infty} \hat{f}_2(y)dy = 0.016$ the area under the girl's weighted higher scoring component and above 238. Thus, by far the largest proportion of higher scoring girls, those with scores above 238, comes from the lower scoring, not the higher scoring component, and in this example, similarly for boys as well.

Keep in mind these probabilities are estimated under the assumption the latent components have normal distributions. The reality may be somewhat different. To repeat, this example illustrates the important fact that higher scoring children come from both mixture components.

One can estimate the number of girls and boys in these upper components by computing $\hat{q}^2 n_g \approx 486$ girls while $\hat{q} n_b \approx 2745$ boys. The X-linked heritability estimate for girls is very small, 0.045, a tiny proportion of total variance for girls: $\widehat{\text{var}}(B_g) + \widehat{\text{var}}(N_g) = 1587.010$ with $\widehat{\text{var}}(B_g) = 70.812$ and $\widehat{\text{var}}(N_g) = 1516.197$. For boys, the X-linked heritability is much larger 0.182, but still relatively small. Thus, the proportion of X-linked variance accounted for in $\mathcal{Y}$ is a small fraction of the total variance for both sexes, a finding entirely expected.

The probability that a given girl's test score y "comes from" the higher scoring second component can also be estimated:

$$\widehat{P}(\text{component } 2 \mid y) = \frac{\hat{q}^2 \hat{f}_2(y)}{\hat{f}_g(y)}.$$

However, to do so requires $f_1(y)$ and $f_2(y)$ to be specified, perhaps as normal distributions.

5.1.3.1 Standard Errors

Standard errors associated with the parameter estimates are reported above in this example because the elements of V seem to have been the result of random sampling assumptions, at least approximately. These standard errors were obtained using the *parametric bootstrap* [27, p. 53], assuming that *post* estimation, the component distributions $f_1(y)$ and $f_2(y)$ are normal in distribution. Whenever standard errors appear, they were obtained by the parametric bootstrap, the components are assumed to be normal, and the elements of V are assumed to be obtained by random sampling, at least approximately.

Standard errors for parameter estimates obtained from large sample survey V, for NAEP or PISA, are not given. For one, there are no sample sizes associated with the estimates in V, and for another, estimates in V are far removed from random sample estimates. These facts were noted in Chap. 2. There is simply no guidance on how one might proceed to construct a standard error for, say, $\hat{q}$ estimated from NAEP data, and thus no standard errors appear.

5.1.4 Example 4: CogAT or Cognitive Abilities Test

The CogAT is a multiple choice test, with varying types of number puzzles, analogies, and series. This example employs an earlier version of the CogAT from 1987 [111] and involved eighth grade children. The observed V which satisfies mdo and predicted $\widehat{V}$ are

$$V = \{101, 100, 16, 14, 5085, 5148\},$$

$$\widehat{V} = \{101, 100, 16.091, 13.896\}.$$

Below are parameter estimates with standard errors in parentheses:

$$\begin{aligned}
\hat{q} &= 0.015(0.008),\\
\hat{q}^2 &= 0.0002(0.0003),\\
\hat{\mu}_1 &= 99.98(0.19),\\
\hat{\mu}_2 &= 166.84(38),\\
\hat{\sigma}^2 &= 192.08(5.6),\\
h^2_{bx} &= 0.258(0.037), \text{ and}\\
h^2_{gx} &= 0.005(0.003).
\end{aligned}$$

The X-linked heritability for girls is vanishing small, but for boys much larger.

Figure 5.2 graphically illustrates this solution, which is very unlike Fig. 5.1. It reveals no clear visual separation between $\hat{f}_b(y)$ and $\hat{f}_g(y)$ nor among the latent component distributions either. That is because $\hat{q} = 0.015$ is very small, so the higher component probability weights for both sexes are near zero, driving these higher scoring components toward zero for all y. Specifically, for girls $\hat{q}^2 \hat{f}_2(y) = 0.0002 \hat{f}_2(y)$, and for boys $\hat{q} \hat{f}_2(y) = 0.015 \hat{f}_2(y)$. Thus, the weighted first component distributions for both sexes and $\hat{f}_b(y)$ and $\hat{f}_g(y)$ all graphically essentially coincide. Some evidence of the second component boys' distribution is just noticeable in the right tail of Fig. 5.2.

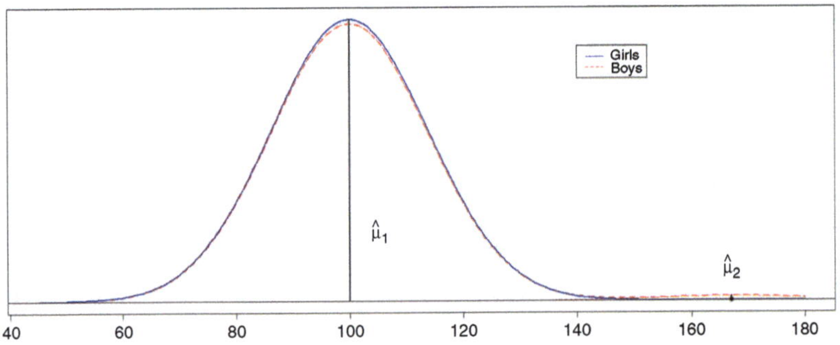

Fig. 5.2 Example 4. Bold lines are $\hat{f}_b(y)$ for boys and $\hat{f}_g(y)$ girls. The second higher component distribution for boys is just graphically distinguishable. The lower scoring component lines merge with the $\hat{f}_b(y)$ and $\hat{f}_g(y)$ distributions and are not graphically distinguishable

Compare the bootstrap standard error associated with $\hat{\mu}_1$ of 0.19 with the standard error associated with $\hat{\mu}_2$ of 38. The uncertainty regarding the location of the second component mean μ_2 is large. That is because there are few observations expected to be in the extreme right tails of the distributions on which to base the location of μ_2 and so the uncertainty with respect to the location of μ_2 is large. One only expects about $1 \approx 0.0002 \times 5{,}148$ girl and about $77 \approx 0.015 \times 5{,}085$ boys in the right higher scoring components.

Even though a glance at Fig. 5.2 suggests there are no sex differences in math, the inequalities in V require an explanation. While $\bar{x}_g$ and $\bar{x}_b$ differ by only one, they are more than three standard errors apart. $\widehat{V}$ is close to V, so $\mathcal{Y}$ provides a coherent explanation, although the sex differences are not evident graphically.

5.1.5 *Example 5: Stone's 1908 Math Tests*

As noted at the outset, Stone [3] constructed two tests: a fundamental test the results of which were displayed in Fig. 1.1 and the other one an arithmetical reasoning test. Both tests were intended for use with sixth grade children. There are 14 numerical fundamental items which assessed addition, subtraction, multiplication, and division. The first of which was the addition of the following numbers (arranged in a column): 2375, 4052, 6345, 260, 5041, and 1543. Problem 14: Multiply 96879 by 896. There were 12 reasoning problems. The first is "If you buy 2 tablets at 7 cents each, and a book for 65 cents, how much change should you receive from a two-dollar bill?" The items of both tests were presented in an increasing order of difficulty, with the sequence determined at least in part, by earlier pretesting. Children were given 12 minutes for the fundamentals and 15 minutes for the reasoning test. The number and ages of children tested were not specified, but comments suggest about 3000 sixth graders received both tests in 26 different school systems.

The scoring for both tests employed item weighting which was based on Thorndike's belief that "arithmetic is but an abstract name for a number of partially independent abilities [3, p. 20]." Weights were designed to reflect the difficulty of the item. The precise way by which weighting was determined seems unclear. In the end, scores for the 12 reasoning items ranged from 0 to 15.2, while for the 14 fundamental items, scores ranged from 0.3 to 6.3.

Stone provided data from 250 boys and 250 girls, "...500 pupils chosen at random from four representative public school systems [3, p. 30]" in his Table X and Table XI. These data, aggregated over the four school systems from his two tables, are given in Table 5.1 for the fundamentals test and in Table 5.2 for the reasoning test. The data from Table 5.1 provided the basis for Fig. 1.1.

Stone's effort was impressive for the time. He had to score, weight items of individual tests, apparently all by hand, with medians replacing means, and Thorndike's AD or average deviation replacing the standard deviation. He credits

Table 5.1 Stone's (1908) Fundamental Data

Score	# Boys	# Girls	Score	# Boys	# Girls
0.3	1	0	3.4	9	8
0.9	0	2	3.5	3	7
1.1	4	2	3.6	3	2
1.2	1	2	3.7	3	1
1.3	2	2	3.8	3	4
1.4	2	4	3.9	6	8
1.5	4	3	4.0	9	6
1.6	2	2	4.1	9	4
1.7	3	3	4.2	4	2
1.8	2	3	4.3	3	1
1.9	10	10	4.4	3	3
2.0	7	10	4.5	4	2
2.1	6	11	4.6	4	4
2.2	3	6	4.7	6	5
2.3	6	9	4.8	4	5
2.4	5	6	4.9	3	4
2.5	4	3	5.0	5	5
2.6	7	7	5.1	1	2
2.7	9	11	5.3	3	1
2.8	7	10	5.4	2	1
2.9	15	15	5.5	2	0
3.0	28	24	5.6	1	0
3.1	9	11	5.8	0	1
3.2	9	6	6.3	1	0
3.3	13	12			

Table 5.2 Stone's (1908) Reasoning Data

Score	# Boys	# Girls	Score	# Boys	# Girls
0	4	5	6.0	3	6
1.0	1	8	6.1	2	2
1.3	1	0	6.2	11	6
1.8	1	0	6.4	29	14
2.0	6	7	6.6	8	11
2.2	0	3	6.8	0	2
2.3	1	1	6.9	1	0
2.4	0	1	7.0	6	3
2.5	0	1	7.1	2	0
2.6	0	1	7.2	2	2
2.8	1	0	7.4	1	1
3.0	12	15	7.5	0	10
3.2	1	2	7.6	20	10
3.3	1	1	7.7	0	1
3.4	1	2	7.8	10	2
3.6	0	4	8.0	7	4
3.7	0	1	8.1	0	1
4.0	12	23	8.2	4	4
4.2	1	2	8.4	0	2
4.3	0	1	8.6	1	2
4.4	2	2	9.2	19	9
4.5	1	0	9.6	2	1
4.6	2	5	9.8	5	0
4.7	0	2	10.0	0	1
4.8	1	2	10.2	5	3
4.9	1	1	11.1	1	1
5.0	20	19	11.2	8	3
5.1	0	1	11.6	1	0
5.2	7	11	12.2	1	0
5.3	0	1	12.7	1	0
5.4	11	17	13.2	1	1
5.6	5	6	14.3	1	0
5.8	3	2	15.2	1	0
5.9	1	1			

his wife for doing much of the statistical analysis. Much of thrust of his work was to compare test performances of different school systems and their relative performance on the two tests. For example, he compares the ratio of boys to girls in their variabilities, using ratios of AD/median which he called a coefficient of variability. Ratios of these quantities defined his variability index. These ratios are reported for smaller numbers of boys and girls for several different school systems.

His fundamental test results satisfy *mo*:

$$V = \{3.193, 3.026, 1.048, 0.996, 250, 250\}$$

with

$$\hat{V} = \{3.193, 3.026, 1.059, 0.984\}$$

close to V. The estimates are

$$\begin{aligned}
\hat{q} &= 0.175, \\
\hat{q}^2 &= 0.031, \\
\hat{\mu}_1 &= 2.991, \\
\hat{\mu}_2 &= 4.147, \\
\hat{\sigma}^2 &= 0.929, \\
h^2_{bx} &= 0.172, \text{ and} \\
h^2_{gx} &= 0.041.
\end{aligned}$$

Figure 5.3 displays the model estimates for Stone's fundamentals test. The higher scoring latent components for both boys and girls are visible in the figure, which resembles Fig. 5.1.

Stone's reasoning test results satisfy *mdo*:

$$V = \{6.486, 5.440, 2.532, 2.316, 250, 250\},$$

while

$$\hat{V} = \{6.486, 5.440, 2.537, 2.312\}.$$

The estimates are

$$\begin{aligned}
\hat{q} &= 0.500, \\
\hat{q}^2 &= 0.250,
\end{aligned}$$

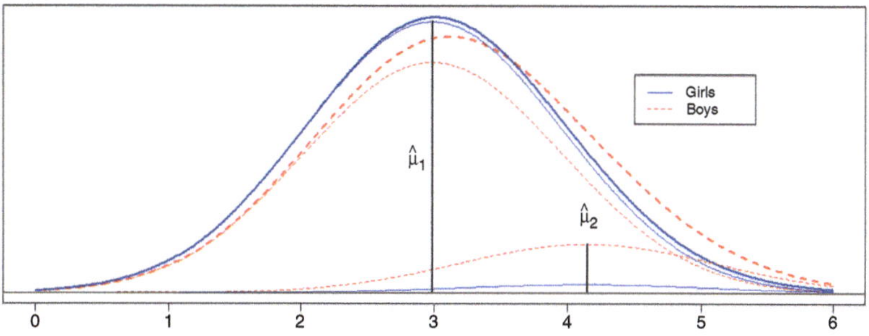

Fig. 5.3 Stone's Fundamentals Test, Example 5, which may be compared with Fig. 1.1

$$\hat{\mu}_1 = 4.393,$$
$$\hat{\mu}_2 = 8.579,$$
$$\hat{\sigma}^2 = 2.057,$$
$$h_{bx}^2 = 0.680, \text{ and}$$
$$h_{gx}^2 = 0.615.$$

The reasoning test estimate of q is far larger than the fundamental test estimate or estimates from the previous two examples. The estimates reflect, of course, weights Stone assigned to each child's test score answer.

Stone stated his primary goal was "...to extract knowledge of the relation between distinctive educational procedures and the resulting products [3, p. 7]." Since his primary interest was in educational procedures, why would he have chosen to provide, as the only raw data tabled, data on boys and girls separately, when numerous other tabulations more central to his stated goal were possible? A speculation is that he observed sex differences in test performance among the 3000 boys and girls he observed in the 26 school systems, in the six chiefly north eastern states he visited; perhaps it was this information he wished to preserve, even though he could not do the analysis he might have wished to do.

5.1.6 Example 6: The Courtis Arithmetic Tests

In 1909, the Russell Sage Foundation of New York City issued a damning report concerning the city's school system "...which indicated that retardation was costing the city millions of dollars annually [112, p. 53]." By any measure, the consequence was extraordinary. A huge investigation was mounted which considered numerous aspects of the educational operation, covering janitorial services, school layout, salaries, teachers' ethnic backgrounds, and more. The concern here is with the only assessment of school achievement, the eight arithmetic tests developed by Stuart A. Courtis. At the time, he was in charge of arithmetic at the Detroit Home and Day School, later the Liggett School, which continues today as the University Liggett School. Later, Courtis joined the University of Michigan as an education professor.

The background and motivation for his tests are set out in five articles spanning the years 1909 to 1911 [113–117]. Subsequent references in this section are all to yet another publication, covering the interval 1911 to 1912 which is the interval Courtis provides for in his report [70]. Courtis constructed all the tests [70, pp. 402-414], supervised the testing and data analysis, and wrote the portion of the final report on testing. It contains more than 150 detailed pages with 50 hand-drawn figures or graphs and 55 tables some spanning multiple pages, with seemingly countless computations, mostly averages. It is a remarkable effort given the limited technology of the period. Interestingly, Courtis declined compensation and received only his expenses [112, p. 58].

Testing involved 33,350 children. The target grades were fourth to eighth, with the addition of two high schools, so data are available through Grade 12. Testing occurred in 903 classes in 52 schools in all five New York city boroughs.

The tests covered basic operations and arithmetic reasoning. Collectively, they were difficult tests. Tests 1 to 4 assessed addition, subtraction, multiplication, and division, respectively, each having 120 items. Test 5 required copying 240 numbers; Tests 6 with 16 items and Test 8 with 8 items were word reasoning tests. Test 7 called fundamentals presented a mixture of arithmetic items requiring all four operations, some very difficult. One item required adding eight five-digit numbers. Children were allowed *one minute* on tests 1 to 6, certainly speed tests. The test forms were labeled as speed tests.

Discussion will focus on those tests which, to varying degrees, clearly address sex differences in performance. These are Tests 1, 3, 6, 7, and 8. *V* can be constructed from data provided by Courtis for one grade level for Test 6 and an aggregate of more than 26,000 children for Test 8. The reasons Tests 6 and 8 can be used for analysis, and not the others, is because they had limited numbers of items, for which exact success frequencies were given. Data for the other tests required grouping the scores into intervals, and in addition, for some intervals data were not available. Testing involved 18 grade levels, 4A and 4B to 12A and 12B, and at each grade level from 1100 to 1200 boys, and a similar number of girls were tested. However, grade level data for both sexes are given only sparingly. One can trust the averages reported. That is because Courtis writes that the averages are aided by "... mechanical tabulation made the average... easily computed [70, p. 432]." AD, average deviations, approximations which replaced standard deviations, followed Thorndike [64].

5.1.6.1 Courtis Tests 1 and 3: Addition and Multiplication

Each test has 120 pairs of single digit numbers, for example, (0, 8) or (2, 5), which were vertically arrayed with answer line below. Items were arranged with six rows of 20 items in each row. For Test 1 children added; for Test 3 they multiplied. Data indicate that in mean, girls generally well exceed boys for both tests at least for the grade levels reported. Data are not reported for all grades and all tests. Data reported are based on the number of items correct for each child. For Test 1, grade 5A girls averaged 49.1, while for boys 47.6 [70, p. 529]. The data are far more convincing for Test 3, multiplication, where averages are given for each sex for eighteen grade levels with means for boys and girls at each grade. In all cases, except for 12B, girls exceed boys in mean [70, p. 525], a fact noted earlier above. At no grade level for Test 3 did the mean exceed 52, less than half the number of items on the test, an indication of the test's difficulty.

5.1.6.2 Courtis Test 6: Simple Reasoning

The first item of this 16 item test reads "The children of a school gave a sleigh-ride party. There were 9 sleighs used, and each sleigh held 30 children. How many children were there in the party? [70, p. 408]." As noted earlier, Lincoln [65, p. 58] shows girls exceed boys at two grades in Test 6 mean, they are tied at three grades, and boys exceed girls at 13 grade levels. A graph [70, p. 527] with mean correct graphed against grade level values 3.5 to grade 12 shows a slightly different Test 6 result with boys exceeding girls at all ages except grade 11.

Courtis provides frequency distributions of scores for Test 6 for grade 7B [70, p. 526] and grade 8A [70, p. 446]; the 8A distribution shows boys with higher mean scores but fails mo. For the 7B data which satisfy mo,

$$V = \{3.714, 3.090, 1.935, 1.823, 1235, 1168\}.$$

Clearly, the test was difficult, with averages less than 4 for a 16 item test.

$$\hat{V} = \{3.714, 3.090, 1.936, 1.822\}$$

$$\begin{aligned} \hat{q} &= 0.487, \\ \hat{q}^2 &= 0.237, \\ \hat{\mu}_1 &= 2.497, \\ \hat{\mu}_2 &= 4.995, \\ \hat{\sigma}^2 &= 2.189, \\ h^2_{bx} &= 0.416, \text{ and} \\ h^2_{gx} &= 0.341. \end{aligned}$$

The estimate of q is quite large and is similar to $\hat{q} = 0.500$ for Stone's reasoning test.

Figures 5.4 and 5.5 display the histograms for boys and girls, respectively. The distributions reveal substantial probability near zero with a sharp bound there. Normal distributions are clearly unsatisfactory as latent distributions because of this sharp lower bound, and hence no latent distributions appear. Both graphs display the location of the estimated component means.

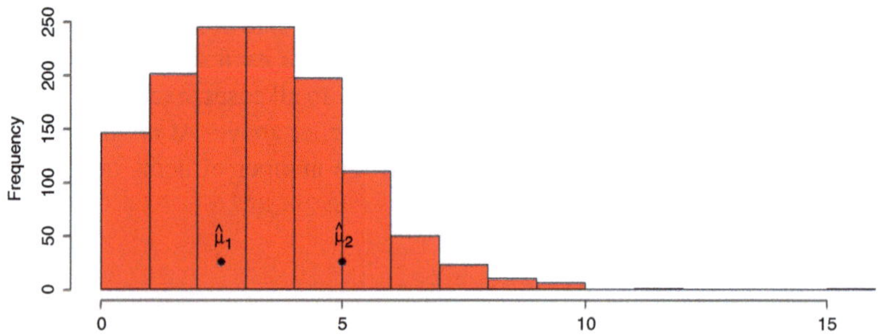

Fig. 5.4 Courtis Reasoning Test 6 histogram for 1,235 boys. Estimated location of component means $\hat{\mu}_1$ and $\hat{\mu}_2$ is shown

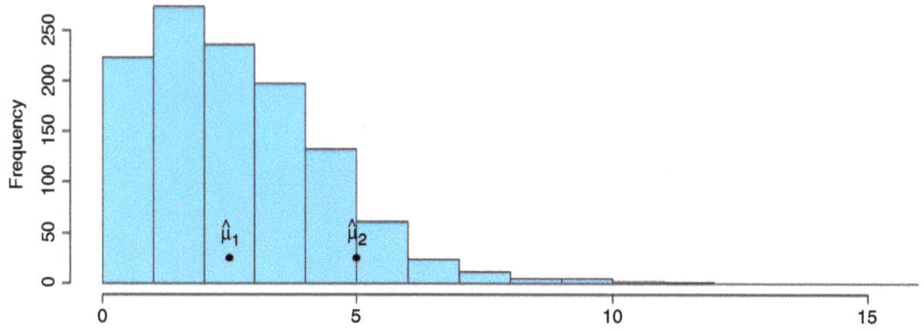

Fig. 5.5 Courtis Reasoning Test 6 histogram for 1,168 girls. Estimated location of component means $\hat{\mu}_1$ and $\hat{\mu}_2$ is shown

5.1.6.3 Courtis Test 7: Fundamentals

This 14 item test [70, p. 410] resembles closely Stone's fundamental test. Test 7 requires mostly multiplication and long division, along with some addition and subtraction problems. The test appears difficult, although children were given 12 minutes. For example, a division item was 3127102÷463, which, by the way, equals 6754. Courtis reports that for grade 8B girls' average correct was 11.1, while boys' average was 10.5 [70, p. 537].

5.1.6.4 Courtis Test 8: Reasoning

Children were allowed six minutes on this eight item word problem test. The first item is "A party of children went from a school to a woods to gather nuts. The number found was but 205, so they bought 1955 nuts more from a farmer. The nuts were shared equally by the children and each received 45. How many children were in the party? [70, p. 414]."

Test scores were integer valued, with possible scores from zero to eight correct. No child, among 27,171 4A through 8B children, correctly answered all eight items. Reported are the corresponding frequencies associated with zero to seven correct [70, p. 531].

$$V = \{0.907, 0.773, 1.069, 0.991, 13629, 13542\}$$

mdo holds; following the analysis

$$\hat{V} = \{0.907, 0.773, 1.070, 0.991\}$$

values which essentially match the observed values. The estimated parameter values are

$$\begin{aligned}\hat{q} &= 0.110,\\ \hat{q}^2 &= 0.012,\\ \hat{\mu}_1 &= 0.756,\\ \hat{\mu}_2 &= 2.132,\\ \hat{\sigma}^2 &= 0.960,\\ h^2_{bx} &= 0.162, \text{ and}\\ h^2_{gx} &= 0.023.\end{aligned}$$

In Figs. 5.6 and 5.7 are histograms for boys and girls, respectively. The modal number correct is zero. Because it is unclear what might be plausible latent discrete component distributions, no estimated distributions are given, but estimated component mean locations are shown.

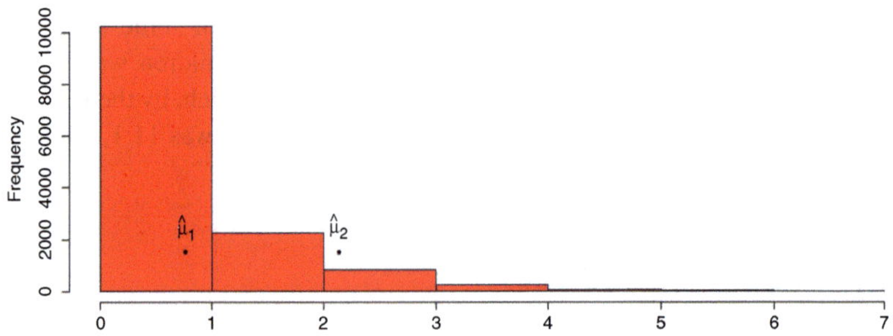

Fig. 5.6 Courtis Reasoning Test 8 Histogram for 13,629 boys. Estimated component locations $\hat{\mu}_1$ and $\hat{\mu}_2$ are shown

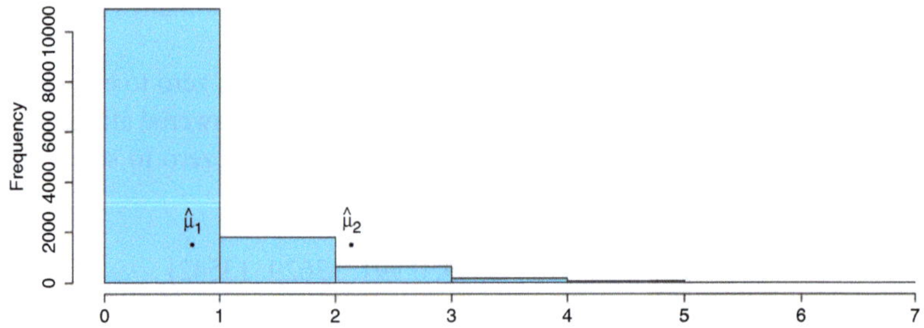

Fig. 5.7 Courtis Reasoning Test 8 Histogram for 13,542 girls. Estimated component locations $\hat{\mu}_1$ and $\hat{\mu}_2$ are shown

5.1.6.5 Courtis Test Summary

"Differences between the abilities of boys and girls there undoubtedly are... [70, p. 524]." The girls exceed boys in multiplication and fall below them in accuracy of work in reasoning. "... the distribution of the individual scores in Tests 3 and 6, which represent the extremes in the amount of difference observed [70, p. 525]." Test 3 is the multiplication test, while Test 6 is the 16 item reasoning test. This result was noted by Lincoln [65, pp. 57–58] and reported in Chap. 2.

Although this work is well more than 100 years old and apparently largely unknown, the care, scope, and effort even by today's standards are impressive. In all cases, children were required to *produce* an answer, so the role of guessing in machine scored multiple choice formats common today is much less of an issue. There was no informed consent back then, and thus the issue of consent's impact on sampling did not occur. One might also imagine that because large-scale testing was not as common earlier on, children would be more attentive and motivated. Courtis' emphasis on test speed was by design. "But by putting the work on a speed basis a situation is created that is much more uniform from individual to individual and from grade to grade... [70, p. 401]." Apparently Courtis directed everything. Today any such effort would have much more dispersed responsibility. One index of the care Courtis exercised is that in recomputing findings from tabled data, only small errors, likely attributed to rounding, have been discovered.

It is worth noting that only a theory would seem to motivate any consideration of why Courtis's data would be interesting to explore from a finite mixture model perspective. Furthermore, only a model that has mixture component distributions unspecified would allow data forming the empirical distributions such as in Figs. 5.6 and 5.7 to be sensibly analyzed.

5.1.7 Example 7: The NAEP Math Tests

The NAEP math tests capture five areas of math content, number properties and operations, measurement, geometry, data analysis and associated statistics and some probability, and algebra, each with varying emphasis at the three grade levels. Millions of children have been tested over the years. In 2019, the test was given to approximately 149,000 grade 4, 147,000 grade 8, and 25,400 grade 12 students [30]. Those NAEP data for estimation are in Tables 2.1 and 2.3. Those years for which V mo is satisfied can provide parameter estimates. Of the 31 possible V, only three eighth grade years fail to satisfy mo. Thus, for grades 4, 8, and 12, there are 13, 10, and 5 estimable V, respectively. The averages of the parameter estimates, with overbars, for each grade are reported below. In parentheses are the standard deviations of the estimates (not standard errors).

5.1.7.1 NAEP Grade Four Math Tests

All 13 V satisfied mdo, with $(s_b^2 - s_g^2)/(\bar{x}_b - \bar{x}_g) \geq 19$ in all cases. The averages of the estimates with the standard deviations of these estimates in parentheses are given below:

$$\begin{aligned}\bar{q} &= 0.044(0.040),\\ \bar{q^2} &= 0.003(0.007),\\ \bar{\mu}_1 &= 232.576(9.505),\\ \bar{\mu}_2 &= 302.719(33.753),\\ \bar{\sigma}^2 &= 850.859(68.895),\\ \bar{h}_{bx}^2 &= 0.118(0.037), \text{ and}\\ \bar{h}_{gx}^2 &= 0.006(0.005).\end{aligned}$$

5.1.7.2 NAEP Grade Eight Math Tests

Of the 13 V 10 satisfy mdo. The averages and standard deviations of the estimates are given below:

$$\begin{aligned}\bar{q} &= 0.020(0.016),\\ \bar{q^2} &= 0.001(0.001),\\ \bar{\mu}_1 &= 276.863(7.150),\\ \bar{\mu}_2 &= 391.887(58.108),\\ \bar{\sigma}^2 &= 1265.758(78.101),\\ \bar{h}_{bx}^2 &= 0.105(0.023), \text{ and}\\ \bar{h}_{gx}^2 &= 0.002(0.001).\end{aligned}$$

5.1.7.3 NAEP Grade Twelve Math Tests

All five V satisfy mdo. And similarly to the above,

$$\begin{aligned}\bar{q} &= 0.047(0.022),\\ \bar{q^2} &= 0.003(0.002),\\ \bar{\mu}_1 &= 150.254(1.475),\\ \bar{\mu}_2 &= 226.013(36.121),\\ \bar{\sigma}^2 &= 1054.533(58.070),\\ \bar{h}_{bx}^2 &= 0.158(0.039), \text{ and}\\ \bar{h}_{gx}^2 &= 0.008(0.002).\end{aligned}$$

5.1.7.4 NAEP Math Tests Summary

The NAEP math test scores in Tables 2.1 and 2.3 are the best estimates of math performance for the general U.S. population of children at three grade levels.

Estimates of q are small, with q^2 vanishingly small for girls. The mean estimates of q at grades four and twelve are nearly identical. The mean X-linked heritabilities $\bar{h}^2_{bx}$ are small and $\bar{h}^2_{gx}$ tiny. Yet the estimates account for the both mean and standard deviation differences between boys and girls in these data. Although not given, $\widehat{V}$ closely match V in all cases. Consequently, there appear few important graphical differences among the different ages or grades. The graph of 2019 grade 12 math solution is displayed below, in Fig. 6.1, to illustrate a related issue.

5.1.8 Example 8: 2003 PISA Math Tests

Table 2.5 provides PISA math V for 41 countries; for five countries mo failed; and these countries appear in bold font. Denmark, Indonesia, and the Netherlands all failed mo because the standard deviations failed to align. In Iceland and Thailand, the mean for girls exceeds the mean for boys. Below are the means of those 36 countries with V satisfying mdo and with corresponding standard deviations of these estimates in parentheses:

$$\begin{aligned}\bar{q} &= 0.135(0.130),\\ \bar{q}^2 &= 0.034(0.056),\\ \bar{\mu}_1 &= 479.315(50.014),\\ \bar{\mu}_2 &= 699.421(274.231),\\ \bar{\sigma}^2 &= 7735.391(1137.271),\\ \bar{h}^2_{bx} &= 0.181(0.067), \text{ and}\\ \bar{h}^2_{gx} &= 0.035(0.044).\end{aligned}$$

Collectively, the influence on X-linkage appears to be greater in these PISA math data than in the U.S. NAEP math data. Here, $\bar{q} = 0.135$. But there is considerable country $\hat{q}$ country variability. Table 5.3 displays in column two the estimates of $\hat{q}$ for math (denoted $\hat{q}_m$) for each country and in columns four and five the estimated heritabilities for boys and girls for math. It will be seen later on that the variability of these $\hat{q}$ seems quite plausible in light of recent paleogenetical studies which upend long held beliefs about the distribution of genes in Europe [118, 119].

Furthermore, the variability of $\hat{q}$ has meaningful associations with different countries' Global Gender Gap Index as will be considered later in Chap. 6. And this diversity, reflected in the variability of $\hat{q}$, might well be expected: "Patterns of genetic diversity have previously been shown to mirror geography on a global scale and within continents and individual countries[120]."

There appear corresponding similarities of PISA math $\hat{q}$ estimates in Table 5.3 related to geography. This matter will be revisited later below, but The Czech Republic with $\hat{q} = 0.302$ and Slovakia with $\hat{q} = 0.351$ have similar large $\hat{q}$ and were a single country until 1993. Finland $\hat{q} = 0.040$ and Sweden $\hat{q} = 0.052$ with far smaller but similar $\hat{q}$ estimates were also a single country until 1809. It is thought these two countries were genetically similar to Norway $\hat{q} = 0.026$ [120].

Table 5.3 PISA Math and Reading Parameter Estimates

Country	$\hat{q}_m$	$\hat{q}_r$	h^2_{bxm}	h^2_{gxm}	h^2_{bxr}	h^2_{gxr}
Australia	0.019	0.461	0.157	0.004	0.617	0.521
Austria	0.037	0.506	0.172	0.008	0.802	0.756
Belgium	0.027	0.410	0.166	0.005	0.436	0.309
Brazil	0.143	0.374	0.199	0.039	0.382	0.241
Canada	0.076	0.404	0.208	0.021	0.480	0.343
Czech Republic	0.302	0.568	0.112	0.047	0.439	0.411
Denmark	NA	0.465	NA	NA	0.322	0.244
Finland	0.040	NA	0.187	0.009	NA	NA
France	0.050	0.470	0.167	0.019	0.586	0.494
Germany	0.068	0.486	0.115	0.009	0.572	0.491
Greece	0.202	0.367	0.243	0.072	0.498	0.333
Hong Kong	0.005	0.327	0.263	0.002	0.549	0.346
Hungary	0.075	0.511	0.096	0.009	0.444	0.382
Iceland	NA	NA	NA	NA	NA	NA
Indonesia	NA	0.614	NA	NA	0.428	0.426
Ireland	0.367	0.534	0.127	0.068	0.446	0.398
Italy	0.144	0.417	0.253	0.053	0.573	0.442
Japan	0.028	0.197	0.229	0.008	0.259	0.076
Korea	0.451	0.462	0.254	0.182	0.261	0.193
Latvia	0.006	0.482	0.160	0.001	0.692	0.616
Lichtenstein	0.247	0.213	0.401	0.171	0.208	0.064
Luxembourg	0.227	0.402	0.187	0.060	0.425	0.294
Macau-China	0.243	0.225	0.295	0.112	0.210	0.068
Mexico	0.193	0.456	0.101	0.025	0.201	0.143
Netherlands	NA	0.477	NA	NA	0.239	0.181
New Zealand	0.148	0.394	0.162	0.032	0.278	0.175
Norway	0.026	0.506	0.167	0.005	0.877	0.845
Poland	0.016	0.448	0.218	0.005	0.637	0.532
Portugal	0.075	0.414	0.250	0.026	0.576	0.443
Russian Federation	0.065	0.329	0.181	0.015	0.386	0.216
Serbia	0.001	NA	0.233	0.000	NA	NA
Slovakia	0.351	0.552	0.170	0.088	0.498	0.460
Spain	0.056	0.464	0.174	0.012	0.632	0.539
Sweden	0.052	0.541	0.093	0.006	0.587	0.543
Switzerland	0.259	0.506	0.143	0.052	0.545	0.477
Thailand	NA	NA	NA	NA	NA	NA
Tunisia	0.476	0.599	0.088	0.063	0.295	0.286
Turkey	0.106	0.388	0.204	0.029	0.479	0.331
United Kingdom	0.087	0.464	0.064	0.006	0.357	0.273
United States	0.025	0.431	0.161	0.005	0.388	0.281
Uruguay	0.145	0.413	0.113	0.021	0.405	0.284

Note: For math, NA denotes *mo* failure. For reading, NA denotes negative $\hat{\sigma}^2$. Subscripts m and r denote math and reading, respectively

In addition, Finland has been an independent country only since 1917 and was largely controlled by the Russian Empire. The Russian Federation with $\hat{q} = 0.065$, given in Table 5.3, seems roughly similar to $\hat{q} = 0.040$ for Finland. Russia and Finland also share a 1340 kilometer border. Geography could be one important reason for similarities of math $\hat{q}$ among some countries.

The estimates of q do, at least in some cases, roughly align with the observed real-world frequencies of behavioral concern. Ceci and Williams observe that "In Turkey, men were overrepresented among computer science graduates by a factor of only 1.79 to 1, while in the Czech Republic, they were overrepresented... by a factor of 6.42 to 1. In the United States the 'male overrepresentation factor' is 2.10 to 1 and in the United Kingdom, 3.10 to 1 [5, p. 168]." The ordering of these countries based on their $\hat{q}$ given in parentheses provides a possible explanation as to why these factors differ:

$$\text{The Czech Republic}(0.302) > \text{Turkey}(0.106) > \text{U.K.}(0.087) > \text{U.S.}(0.025).$$

Only Turkey seems wrongly ordered, given the quote above. Given the interest of the over representation of men in computer science, it is interesting to compare the graphically portrayed solutions of The Czech Republic and the U.S.A.

Figure 5.8 displays the Czech Republic, while Fig. 5.9 displays the U.S.A. The lower component estimated $\hat{\mu}_1$ is similar in their location for the two countries, but for the U.S.A. $\hat{\mu}_2$ is more extremely situated and the upper component is much smaller in size. With the scale of Fig. 5.9, the girls' higher scoring component does not appear in the U.S. graph. In The Czech Republic Fig. 5.8, the higher scoring component is much larger for both boys and girls. The graphical comparisons of the two countries, and the ratio of the boys' Czech Republic's second higher scoring component weight $\hat{q}$ to the corresponding U.S. $\hat{q}$, $0.302/0.025 = 12.08$, would seem to give some indication as to why the computer science graduates in The Czech Republic are far more overrepresented by men than in the U.S.A.

Also, there appears to be evidence of some agreement in the sizes of $\hat{q}$ with estimates from other sources. The U.S. $\hat{q} = 0.025$ is within the range of the

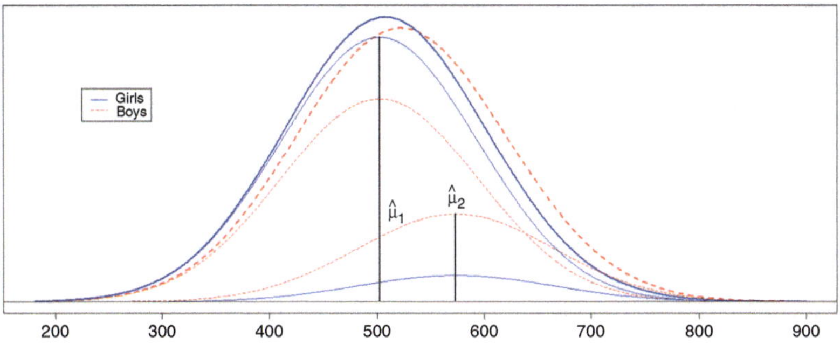

Fig. 5.8 The Czech Republic PISA Math Test Estimated Solution from V in Table 2.5

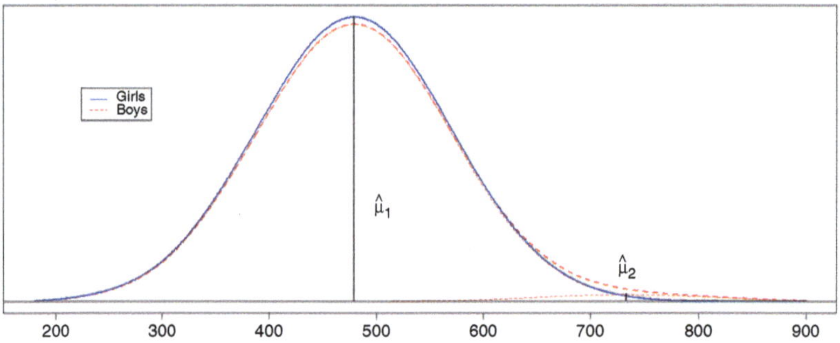

Fig. 5.9 United States PISA Math Test Estimated Solution from V in Table 2.5

corresponding average estimates from NAEP data in Example 7, 0.020 to 0.047. The U.S estimate is also the fifth smallest value among the 36 $\hat{q}$ estimates. So, the U.S. $\hat{q}$ is not large in comparison to mostly European countries. Another example is Italy. From Example 3, $\hat{q} = 0.178$ for Italian children. The PISA estimate for Italy is $\hat{q} = 0.144$.

Just how different are the boys' and girls' math test score distributions in different countries? And just how different are the U.S. boys' and girls' distributions relative to many other countries? The answer is that U.S. boys' and girls' distributions are far more similar than most of the OECD countries. Estimates of the probability distributions $f_b(y)$ and $f_g(y)$ are easily obtained for each country for which mo is satisfied, by replacing that country's parameters with their estimates in their distributions and obtaining estimates $\hat{f}_b(y)$ and $\hat{f}_g(y)$. Once available, an estimate of the Hellinger distance, $\widehat{H}$, defined above, is most easily obtained using numerical integration.

Table 5.4 provides, in column two, $\widehat{Hd} = 100\widehat{H}$ in math for all 41 countries. For those countries for which mo failures occurred, $\widehat{Hd}$ based on normality is given and appear underlined. When $\widehat{Hd}$ is computed under normality, the estimates tend to be somewhat smaller than $\widehat{Hd}$ under $\mathcal{Y}$. There is a sizable range of $\widehat{Hd}$ differences among countries. The U.S. estimated solution displayed in Fig. 5.9 has $\widehat{Hd} = 5.833$.

Macau-China is the second largest among 41 $\widehat{Hd}$ with $\widehat{Hd} = 9.956$ and its corresponding $\hat{q} = 0.243$ is nearly ten times the size of $\hat{q} = 0.025$ for the U.S.A., with estimates given in Table 5.3. Macau-China's graphical solution is given in Fig. 5.10, which shows dramatically the much larger sex differences favoring boys in PISA upper tail math performance than for the U.S.A. Comparing math sex differences in the U.S.A. with other countries reveals that the U.S.A. displays among the smaller sex differences in math test performance as gauged by $\widehat{Hd}$. It is twelfth smallest among those 36 countries with model-based $\widehat{Hd}$ estimates (not underlined) in Table 5.4. As will be seen, much the same situation holds for reading as well except that girls dominate boys.

Table 5.4 PISA $\widehat{Hd}$ and Global Gender Gap Index

Country	$\widehat{Hd}_m$	$\widehat{Hd}_r$	GGGI
Australia	6.075	15.645	0.738
Austria	6.020	17.744	0.781
Belgium	6.874	12.873	0.793
Brazil	9.479	13.523	0.696
Canada	7.027	13.630	0.772
Czech Republic	5.808	12.145	0.710
Denmark	6.441	10.624	0.764
Finland	6.419	20.562	0.860
France	5.810	15.096	0.791
Germany	4.482	14.787	0.801
Greece	8.618	14.108	0.689
Hong Kong	5.291	15.048	NA
Hungary	3.858	12.573	0.699
Iceland	8.046	22.506	0.908
Indonesia	2.031	11.650	0.697
Ireland	6.341	12.476	0.804
Italy	8.505	15.189	0.720
Japan	8.184	9.069	0.650
Korea	9.342	9.458	0.689
Latvia	5.209	16.613	0.771
Lichtenstein	12.294	7.835	NA
Luxembourg	7.402	12.670	0.736
Macau-China	9.956	7.933	NA
Mexico	5.252	8.687	0.764
Netherlands	1.956	8.974	0.767
New Zealand	6.347	9.902	0.841
Norway	5.991	18.281	0.845
Poland	7.156	16.046	0.709
Portugal	8.011	15.239	0.766
Russian Federation	6.198	12.070	NA
Serbia	1.993	20.117	0.779
Slovakia	7.422	13.173	0.717
Spain	5.958	15.866	0.788
Sweden	3.611	14.606	0.822
Switzerland	6.512	14.217	0.795
Thailand	0.030	20.177	0.709
Tunisia	5.936	10.303	0.643
Turkey	7.453	13.695	0.639
United Kingdom	3.010	11.263	0.780
United States	5.833	11.922	0.769
Uruguay	5.405	13.501	0.711

Note: $\widehat{Hd}_m$ is math, and $\widehat{Hd}_r$ is reading. Underlines are estimates under normality. NA = Not Available

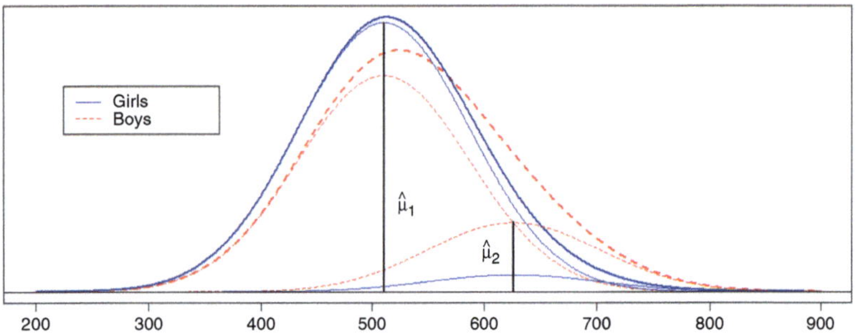

Fig. 5.10 Macau-China PISA Math Test estimated solution from V in Table 2.5

5.2 Reading Examples

The reading V and their corresponding model estimates may be viewed just as the math estimates were viewed. The only fundamental data difference is that $\bar{x}_g > \bar{x}_b$ and associated figures showing boys anchor the bottom of the reading test distributions.

5.2.1 *Example 9: British Reading Test*

Children aged 10 years completed the British reading test called Group Reading Test II [50].

$$V = \{97.50, 100.96, 13.20, 11.58, 117, 115\},$$

which satisfies rdo and with

$$\widehat{V} = \{97.50, 101.00, 13.41, 11.33\}.$$

Below are the parameter estimates, with standard errors in parentheses:

$$\begin{aligned}
\hat{q} &= 0.218(0.16),\\
\hat{q}^2 &= 0.048(0.09),\\
\hat{\mu}_1 &= 81.63(23),\\
\hat{\mu}_2 &= 101.92(49),\\
\hat{\sigma}^2 &= 109.68(30),\\
h_{bx}^2 &= 0.390(0.10), \text{ and}\\
h_{gx}^2 &= 0.145(0.08).
\end{aligned}$$

The estimated higher scoring component, $\hat{f}_2(y)$, has weights $1 - \hat{q} = 0.782$ for boys and $1 - \hat{q}^2 = 0.952$ for girls. The estimated $\widehat{V}$ agrees well with V.

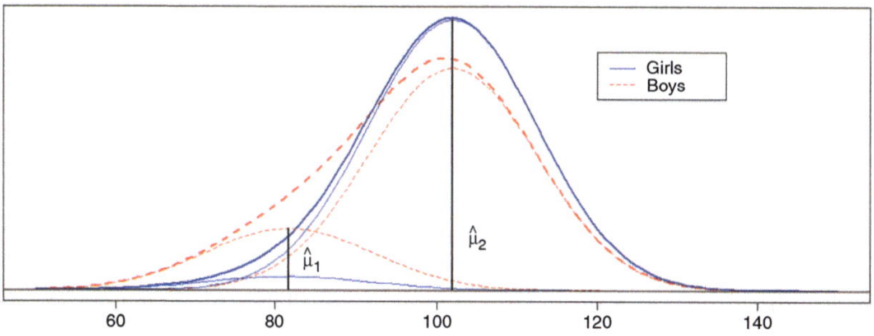

Fig. 5.11 Example 9. Thick lines are $\hat{f}_b(y)$ for boys and $\hat{f}_g(y)$ girls, and thin lines are their two components $\hat{f}_k(y)$ with ordinates at $\hat{\mu}_1$ and $\hat{\mu}_2$ at the estimated means of the two-component densities

Figure 5.11 graphs the estimated solution assuming normal components and displays the estimated component means $\hat{\mu}_1$ and $\hat{\mu}_2$. Notable is the very large excess of boys, relative to girls in the lower tails of their associated distributions. The figure clearly reveals why the reading sample mean for boys is smaller, but sample variance for boys is larger; their upper tails show more similarities. There are more girls than boys in the upper tail regions, although the sizes of the differences are smaller, vanishing so as test scores increase.

5.2.2 *Example 10: The NAEP Reading Tests*

As with the math tests, millions of children have been tested over time. The reading test resembles in spirit many earlier reading tests. There are paragraphs to read which are followed with questions which target three cognitive categories: locate/recall, integrate/interpret, and critique/evaluate, questions that presumably reflect the kinds of thinking required to understand written text. The V data employed are in Tables 2.2 and 2.4. There are 35 reading V; five V fail to satisfy ro, all with standard deviations for boys and girls matching. All 30 V which satisfy ro also satisfy rdo. The mean of the estimates for each grade along with the standard deviation of the estimates in parentheses is given below.

5.2.2.1 NAEP Fourth Grade Reading Tests

The model estimates of 11 V with standard deviations of the estimates in parentheses are given below:

$$\bar{q} = 0.326(0.083),$$
$$\bar{q}^2 = 0.112(0.055),$$
$$\bar{\mu}_1 = 192.320(6.651),$$

$$\begin{aligned}\bar{\mu}_2 &= 227.152(1.733),\\ \bar{\sigma}^2 &= 1200.524(90.431),\\ \bar{h}^2_{bx} &= 0.178(0.058), \text{ and}\\ \bar{h}^2_{gx} &= 0.091(0.054).\end{aligned}$$

5.2.2.2 NAEP Eighth Grade Reading Tests

As above, the estimates of the 12 V and their standard deviations in parentheses are given

$$\begin{aligned}\bar{q} &= 0.507(0.044),\\ \bar{q}^2 &= 0.259(0.044),\\ \bar{\mu}_1 &= 236.431(6.143),\\ \bar{\mu}_2 &= 280.423(2.884),\\ \bar{\sigma}^2 &= 777.853(160.755),\\ \bar{h}^2_{bx} &= 0.385(0.136), \text{ and}\\ \bar{h}^2_{gx} &= 0.329(0.141).\end{aligned}$$

5.2.2.3 NAEP Twelfth Grade Reading Tests

With seven V, the estimates and corresponding standard deviations in parentheses are given below:

$$\begin{aligned}\bar{q} &= 0.474(0.098),\\ \bar{q}^2 &= 0.233(0.091),\\ \bar{\mu}_1 &= 255.198(2.288),\\ \bar{\mu}_2 &= 307.203(8.360),\\ \bar{\sigma}^2 &= 775.978(408.644),\\ \bar{h}^2_{bx} &= 0.488(0.239), \text{ and}\\ \bar{h}^2_{gx} &= 0.417(0.280).\end{aligned}$$

5.2.2.4 NAEP Reading Test Analysis Summary

As with math, although not displayed, $\widehat{V}$ closely resemble V in all cases, in many cases matching V, as do all twelfth grade $\widehat{V}$. The estimates of q for reading are much larger than estimates of q for math. The much larger mean separation favoring girls in reading reflects the much larger $\hat{q}$ estimates. Heritabilities are larger as well, with average X-linked heritabilities increasing with age, for both boys and girls, a commonly observed finding with polygene heritability estimates.

Figure 5.12 shows the graphic for the 2015 grade 12 NAEP reading V in Table 2.4. As with the previous example, it reflects the often observed commentary in the literature, namely there are more girls in their upper tail than there are boys

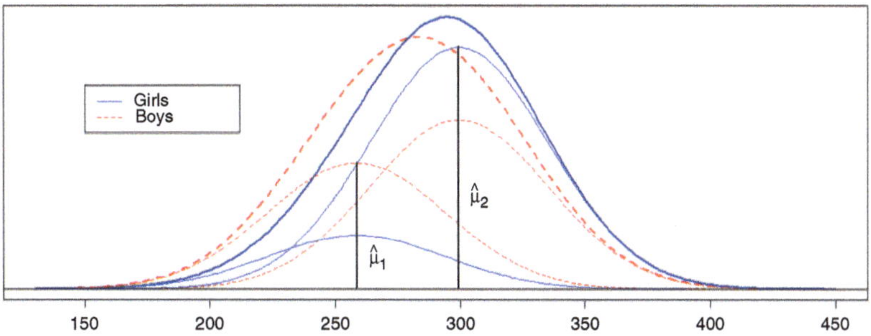

Fig. 5.12 NAEP 2015 grade 12 reading estimated solution, V from Table 2.4. Thick lines are $\hat{f}_b(y)$ for boys and $\hat{f}_g(y)$ girls, and thin lines are their two components $\hat{f}_k(y)$ with ordinates at $\hat{\mu}_1$ and $\hat{\mu}_2$ at the estimated means of the two component densities

in their upper tail of the reading test score distributions, but more boys than girls in the lower tail regions as have been reported [121, 122].

Focusing on Fig. 5.12, the probability area between the solid and dashed bold lines can be estimated under $\mathcal{Y}$ for intervals of interest. The equations of concern are all defined in Chap. 4. For example, $\int_{300}^{\infty}[\hat{f}_g(y) - \hat{f}_b(y)]dy = 0.091$. So, there are about 9% more girls in this upper tail region above 300 than there are boys. The solid and dashed bold lines cross in Fig. 5.12 at reading score 279. The area difference between the corresponding boys and girls lower tails is, up to the point where the dashed and solid bold lines cross, $\int_{-\infty}^{279}[\hat{f}_b(y) - \hat{f}_g(y)]dy = 0.106$ reflecting the obvious excess of boys relative to girls in the lower tail regions, here about 11%.

5.2.3 Example 11: 2003 PISA Reading Tests

Table 2.6 provides the PISA reading V for 41 countries. Compared with the different countries mean math sex differences, the reading mean differences are much larger. The reading differences $\bar{x}_g - \bar{x}_b$ range from 13.27 to 57.76. By comparison, $\bar{x}_b - \bar{x}_g$ for math range from -15.41 to 28.84. The average of the 39 mean math differences favoring boys is 10.313. The average of all 41 reading differences favoring girls $\mathcal{Y}$ is a random effects model, and 33.682.

Although all countries well satisfied rdo, four V failed in parameter estimation: Finland, Iceland, Serbia, and Thailand. These countries have large mean separation, always more than 42 points. $\mathcal{Y}$ is the random effects model, and σ^2 is estimated by a subtraction. Consequently, the estimate can be negative. $\hat{\sigma}^2$ was negative for these four countries and so parameter estimation under $\mathcal{Y}$ failed. Parameter estimates are available for 37 countries. Below are the means of the 37 countries' estimates, with the standard deviations of the estimates in parentheses:

$$\begin{aligned}
\bar{q} &= 0.440(0.096),\\
\bar{q}^2 &= 0.203(0.080),\\
\bar{\mu}_1 &= 390.983(44.857),\\
\bar{\mu}_2 &= 525.916(44.305),\\
\bar{\sigma}^2 &= 5190.130(2701.927),\\
\bar{h}^2_{bx} &= 0.460(0.271), \text{ and}\\
\bar{h}^2_{gx} &= 0.364(0.316).
\end{aligned}$$

The sizes of these much larger sex differences in reading are attributable to much larger estimates of q and thus q^2 for reading than the smaller q and often vanishing q^2 estimated values for math. The reading $\hat{q}$ (denoted as $\hat{q}_r$) are given in column three of Table 5.3, along with X-linked estimated reading heritabilities in columns six and seven. $\widehat{Hd}$ for reading are given in column three of Table 5.4. For those countries where estimation failed, *Hd* estimates under normality are given and denoted by underline. There are large differences between boys' and girls' reading distributions among the countries and typically far larger than the math differences as may be seen by comparing columns two and three in Table 5.4. As with math, the reading distributional differences for the U.S.A. are comparatively small, with the U.S. distributional difference $\widehat{Hd} = 11.922$ the twelfth smallest of the 37 model-based *Hd* estimates.

Pictorially, the contrast is illustrated in Figs. 5.13 and 5.14 which gives the graphs of the countries with the smallest and largest $\mathcal{Y}$-based estimates $\widehat{Hd}$. Liechtenstein has the smallest separation, with $\widehat{Hd} = 7.835$ and Norway with $\widehat{Hd} = 18.281$ the largest (again, among those countries without their $\widehat{Hd}$ underlined in column three of Table 5.4).

The graph for Norway might seem implausibly surreal with a clear estimated bimodality in reading scores for both boys and girls. In the PIRLS Norway reading data [14, Table 3] for the 2001 and 2006 assessment cycles, both V satisfy rdo and yield graphs more like Fig. 5.11, without the clear bimodal of Fig. 5.14. However, it

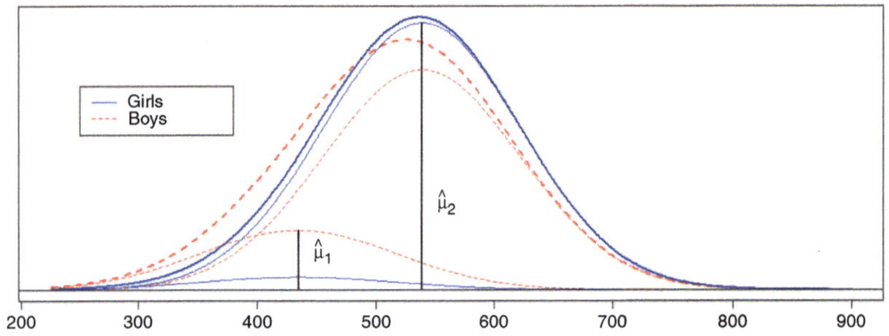

Fig. 5.13 Liechtenstein PISA reading solution, V data from Table 2.6. Thick lines are $\hat{f}_b(y)$ for boys and $\hat{f}_g(y)$ girls, and thin lines are their two components $\hat{f}_k(y)$ with ordinates at $\hat{\mu}_1$ and $\hat{\mu}_2$ at the estimated means of the two component densities

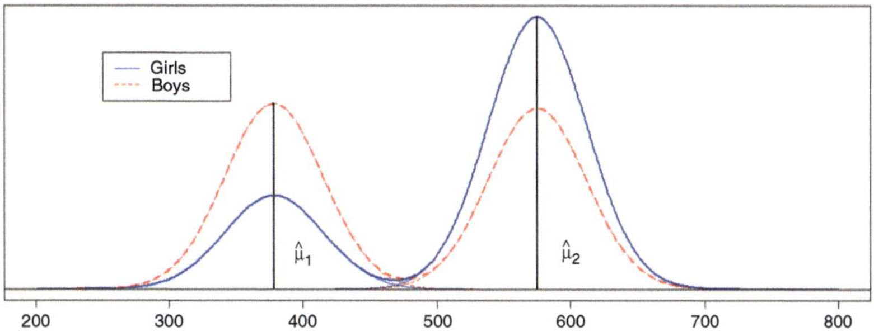

Fig. 5.14 Norway PISA reading solution, V from Table 2.6. The distributions $\hat{f}_b(y)$ for boys and $\hat{f}_g(y)$ girls coincide with their component distributions $\hat{f}_1(y)$ and $\hat{f}_2(y)$ because the components are widely separated. The standard deviation of each component is 37, while the component means $\hat{\mu}_1$ and $\hat{\mu}_2$ are 197 points apart. Thus, the component means are more than five standard deviations apart

is expected boys and girls, in some countries, would reveal bimodal test performance even in smaller samples, given the sizes of the reading test performance differences in some countries. The 2006 PIRLS V for Qatar [14, Table 3] yields graphical bimodalities under $\mathcal{Y}$.

It is difficult to overemphasize how much girls dominate boys in reading, seemingly in all developed countries worldwide. However, the database here considers largely OECD countries, those with PISA scores. The sizes of reading mean differences favoring girls simply far exceed the size by which boys typically exceed girls in math test mean.

Chapter 6
Summaries and Model Extensions

Further model applications, analytical extensions, and clarifications are detailed in 12 sections after the first section which summarizes results and implications of the Chap. 5 analyses.

6.1 Empirical and Conceptual Main Points

It seems reasonable to suspect that anyone who has read this far is likely to be much more interested in sex differences in math than in sex differences in reading. One might therefore start on a lighter note by observing that perhaps the above theory might provide the justification for a popular book's title: *The Math Gene* [123]. Curiously, the title is misleading. Devlin rejects any notion of a math gene. He writes "Roughly speaking, by 'the math gene' I mean 'an innate facility for mathematical thought... ' [123, p. xvi]."

"There *cannot* be any single or simple answer to the many complex questions about sex differences in math and science. Readers expecting a single conclusion...are surely disappointed [12, p. 41, italics added]." Ignoring the arrogance of the claim, certainly there are settings in which sex differences concerning math and science are boldly evident and which may be the result of bias or discrimination [124]. Such matters are certainly of concern. However, one of the most important, most widely noted, and most puzzling sex differences has concerned differences in math test score distributions obtained in observational settings. Such distributional differences have been evident for more than a century in the U.S.A. and are evident globally today. These differences have now been coherently explained by a model which, at root, is little more than the model for two independent coin flips. All the analytical model inequalities can be traced to sex differences in probabilistic outcomes of binary events. The same model addresses the widely neglected but far larger sex differences in reading test score distributions as well.

H. Thomas, *Sex Differences in Reading and Math Test Scores of Children*, Monographs in the Psychology of Education,
https://doi.org/10.1007/978-3-031-41272-1_6

Thus, contrary to what has been claimed (with some exceptions to be addressed momentarily), a simple and coherent answer *can* be given to empirical test score sex differences puzzles. It is simply a matter of first, recognizing the patterns in data, as Kagan [34] wisely stressed, and second, modeling the processes appropriately. The answer provided by $\mathcal{Y}$ may not be a popular answer, nor perhaps the answer hoped for or desired. However, $\mathcal{Y}$ provides a plausible answer. There exists no alternative, formal, or otherwise, which provides the conceptual basis for addressing a wide range of empirical facts and in particular provides the theoretical basis for the inequalities of $\mathcal{S}$. The level of model to empirical correspondence, that is, the correspondence between V and $\widehat{V}$ especially within a simple framework, seems rare. Consequently, it seems reasonable to suggest that $\mathcal{Y}$ resembles the process that generated the V sample data. $\mathcal{Y}$ has just three critical parameters to estimate: $q, \mu_2 - \mu_1$, and σ, the same number as the effect size δ. If the law of parsimony (Occam's razor) applies, then $\mathcal{Y}$ would appear to set a high bar for alternative explanations to achieve. Any competing framework must coherently account for the inequalities of $\mathcal{S}$ and hope to do so with three parameters.

There are settings where $\mathcal{Y}$ does not hold, or at least the estimation algorithm fails, even if the elements of $\mathcal{S}$ are satisfied. In the case of PISA math testing, in five countries mo fails. These countries are noted in Table 2.5. In some cases, these failures may be because of sampling variation when q for math for a particular country may be small. It may be because of girls' dominant advantage in reading, thus facilitating girls' performance on some PISA math test items. The language of the country in which the test is administered may impact boys and girls differently, thus influencing math test performance in ways not fully understood. And it must be admitted that the model may be flat-out wrong, at least for some countries.

For reading scores, rdo seems to nearly invariably hold, and PISA test failures of four countries in Table 2.6, and noted in Sect. 5.2.3 were of a different kind, namely estimation failures when $\hat{\sigma}^2 < 0$. It seems likely the assumption that N_b and N_g share the same variance is wrong. There are several cases as well where mdo holds, but estimation fails for example [47], and likely for the same reason. Relaxing the equal variance assumption could be addressed within a likelihood model framework, but estimation in this case would require a data stream, much more conceptual machinery, and iterative methods.

While there are no competing models to $\mathcal{Y}$, no claim is made that the model is the "correct" model as all models are wrong models [125]. However, even wrong models can be useful, and the breadth of explanatory power seems remarkable for simple model. The model appears to provide a coherent explanation for the widely noted differences among countries in their PISA test scores, except for those cases just mentioned. Being able to estimate the parameters of $\mathcal{Y}$ based on elements of V without requiring a raw data stream and then subsequently being able to illustrate the model graphically can certainly be viewed as a model strength. There are numerous other V which could be analyzed. What has been presented is only a sampling.

It has been noted repeatedly that the estimates of q for math are generally small and correspondingly so are the X-linked heritabilities for math for both boys and girls. This result reveals that most of the test score variance in data is unexplained, an outcome that was expected. X-linked heritabilities are far larger for reading, but substantial variance remains unaccounted in reading test scores as well. Thus, there is much research required to identify other plausible and likely larger sources of variance.

To untangle other sources of influence is likely to require new frameworks for thinking about sex differences which puts empirical regularities at the center of attention as, to note again, Kagan [34] has eloquently argued. This simply has not occurred. Witness the general disregard for differences in test score variances as having any substantive relevance for understanding either math or reading test score sex differences. The viewpoint here is that effect size approaches have hijacked efforts at understanding and impeded if not halted conceptual progress. Meta-analysis approaches have not contributed to conceptual understanding, a fact that has long been recognized [126]. Yet the belief in the value of effect size analysis has grown such that it is has been claimed it is a viable framework for *any* sex difference variables of interest.

In Figure 1 [15] are displayed four panels. In each panel are two equal variance but shifted normal distributions; each panel implies a different effect size. The authors write "Figure 1 shows four possible alternatives for the distribution of males' and females' scores on a trait, which could be *anything* from hippocampus size to mathematics performance [15, p. 177, italics added]." Such a statement implies a remarkably naive belief that all between-group mean differences are understandable through a location-shift, effect size framework, as if this perspective is the only way by which Nature could produce sex differences in task performance.

Not only is an effect size approach inappropriate for math (and reading) test scores, but it is inappropriate for the measures of the hippocampus as well. That is because, while it might be surprising to learn, *mo* holds for hippocampus volumes as well. Ritchie and others in their Table 1 [127] report the means and standard deviations of the left and right hippocampus volumes of 2466 men and 2750 women. Data for both left and right volumes satisfy *mo* as do *all 15 additional* brain variables in their table.

Two cognitive test variables reporting sex differences also appear in their Table 1. One test satisfies *mo*, while the other test reports reaction times. Perhaps the questions should be, first, for what sex difference variables is an effect size model δ appropriate and thus the calculation of d sensible? Second, could X-linkage play a role in brain sex differences?

Nature can produce sex differences in test score distributions, or sex differences in other settings, by many different vehicles. The researcher's task is to attempt to learn which vehicle Nature uses and to try to model that process suitably. This fundamental step in the research process has gone missing.

Under $\mathcal{Y}$, it is assumed Nature produces distributional differences by a *frequency* mechanism which is different from a *location-shift* mechanism. This is illustrated by all the Chap. 5 examples. Recall that under $\mathcal{Y}$ both boys and girls share identical latent component distributions, $f_k(y), k = 1, 2$, so boys and girls within the same component share identical math test score distributions. What produces the mean differences (and variance differences) are the frequencies with which these scores appear. These frequency differences are determined by the component coefficients, functions of q and q^2. Another way of thinking about differences, and as noted earlier, is that $\mathcal{Y}$ models the latent within-sex differences, and these within-sex differences produce the between-sex differences observed in data. By understanding within-sex differences, the between-sex observed differences may well take care of themselves [128].

"This book is about the reasons males are overrepresented in mathematics and mathematically intensive professions... [5, p. ix]." This was the motivation of Ceci and Williams, 2010. Their motivation was clearly a frequency matter, not a location-shift matter: why are there more men than women in some professions? Yet in "Gauging the size of sex differences," they use d [5, pp. 20–21] which does not index frequency differences. This does not imply of course that a location-shift perspective cannot often lead, plausibly, to observed frequency differences. But given that interest in sex differences often starts with everyday observations of frequency differences of boys and girls or men and women in various settings [23], it does suggest that one needs a broader perspective in how sex differences are conceptualized. Although it may seem heretical to suggest it, abandoning the devotion to effect sizes may be a good place to start. There is much to admire about the openness and scholarly approach of the now rarely referenced nearly 50 year old Maccoby and Jacklin book [53].

Recently, Casey and Ganley [20] have expressed interest in considering within sex differences. Latent processes often viewed as latent distributions appear to have attracted little interest among sex differences researchers. The main reason is likely because of the dominance of effect size procedures which leave no space for latent variables thinking achievable through mixture models [99, 129]. If between-group differences are the result of within-group component distributions with different component weights, as in $\mathcal{Y}$, then no between-group location-shift model is appropriate. That is because each group's probability distribution is of a different shape. Under a location-shift perspective, the distributions of different groups remain identical in shape. In real-world realizations, however, there may appear to be no sex differences in graphical portrayals as Fig. 5.2 of Example 4 reveals.

One conceptual fact that needs to be emphasized and was described in Example 3 and illustrated in Fig. 5.1. Namely, that for both sexes, the majority of high math performers come from the lower, not higher scoring latent component. This is true for example, for the U.S. PISA math data, portrayed in Fig. 5.9. Only those boys with scores above 667 more probably come from the higher component. Virtually all higher scoring girls come from the lower scoring component. The reason is because both for boys and girls the proportions of individuals in the higher scoring component are small, so most of the probability mass is in the lower scoring PISA math component. For boys the higher scoring component has about 2.5% of the total probability mass, while for girls it is about 0.1%.

To maintain the view that, under $\mathcal{Y}$, only those boys and girls in the higher scoring components are high math achievers—which a casual reader might believe—is incorrect. An interesting question to ponder, however, is whether two individuals with the same high math score, but with scores that arise from different latent component distributions, are equally talented.

$\mathcal{Y}$ has nearly 40-year old conceptual roots [104]. There is a historical commentary about this early work and its corresponding reception [130]. The following 12 sections address additional model applications, add some further analytical results, and consider issues which have been alluded to earlier.

6.2 Math Meta-analyses and Variance Ratios

The puzzle of why small $d > 0$ and small average d or $\bar{d} > 0$ are commonly observed in math meta-analyses was noted at the outset in Chap. 1. No conceptual interpretation of these findings has appeared. However, from the perspective of $\mathcal{Y}$, a conceptual explanation emerges.

To see how d is viewed under $\mathcal{Y}$, replace the sample values in the expression for d, given at the outset in Chap. 1 with their $\mathcal{Y}$ parameter values, given in Chap. 4. For example, replace $\bar{x}_b$ with $\mu_b = q(1-q)\mu_1 + q\mu_2$ and s_g^2 with $\sigma_g^2 = q^2(1-q)^2(\mu_2 - \mu_1)^2 + \sigma^2$. After some algebra, obtain

$$\eta = \frac{q(1-q)}{\sqrt{1/\xi^2 + q(1-q^3)/2}}$$

with $\xi = (\mu_2 - \mu_1)/\sigma$. Thus, d under $\mathcal{Y}$ estimates η, not δ, and η provides the conceptual model for d under $\mathcal{Y}$.

Although η has no useful math-substantive interpretation, inspection of η reveals why small $d > 0$ appear. First, $\eta > 0$, so $d > 0$ are expected. Second, η will be small when q is small, and estimates $\hat{q}$ suggest q for math is small—at least for U.S. math test results. Hence, $d > 0$ should be small. As $q \to 0$, $\eta \to 0$ and similarly for d. η increases with increasing component mean difference $\mu_2 - \mu_1$. η increases with decreasing σ and correspondingly increasing ξ. $\eta \in (0, 0.556)$ and is maximum when $\xi = \infty$ and $q \approx 0.37$.

For illustration, consider Example 4. $d = 0.067$; replacing the parameters in η with estimates gives $\hat{\eta} = 0.067$ with $\hat{q} = 0.015$. Of course, d will not always be positive, but in expectation under $\mathcal{Y}$ it should be. Thus, $\mathcal{Y}$ provides an explanation revealing why small $d > 0$ appear and in particular small $\bar{d} > 0$ in math meta-analyses.

Variance ratios of s_b^2/s_g^2 greater than one have also been a puzzle. As with the above, replace the sample quantities with the quantities which they estimate under $\mathcal{Y}$, and then form the corresponding ratio. s_b^2/s_g^2 estimates the ratio σ_b^2/σ_g^2 which equals

$$\frac{q(1-q)(\mu_2 - \mu_1)^2 + \sigma^2}{q^2(1-q^2)(\mu_2 - \mu_1)^2 + \sigma^2}.$$

Inspection reveals why the corresponding sample ratios are larger than one. That is because $q(1-q) > q^2(1-q^2)$ when $0 < q < 0.618$. Estimates of $\hat{q}$ have been well less than 0.618 for both reading and math. For Example 4, $s_b^2/s_g^2 = 1.306$, while the model expression, just above, with estimates replacing parameters gives 1.341.

6.3 Arguments Against Genetic Influences

It is difficult to find explicit statements as to why sex differences, especially in math, are not to be found in matters genetic. But consider these quotes:

> For some countries, girls do as well or better than boys at the left tail, but worse at the right tail (United States, Hungary). In other countries, sex differences are most pronounced in the middle of the distribution (Russia, Austria). It is hard to come up with a compelling genetic explanation for such diversity! [5, p. 164].

> If the genetic contribution were strong, however, then males should predominate at the upper tail of performance in all countries and at all times, and the male-female ratio should be of comparable size across different samples [131, p. 956].

> ...there is no reason to believe that the genetic factors involved in determining gender will vary across countries, implying that to the degree that gender differences in mathematics result from genetic factors, there should be no international variation in these differences [132, p. S140].

> ...the gender gap in math differs substantially across countries. Hence, 'nature' cannot be the only account for the females' disadvantage in math; there must be alternative explanations...[61, p. 2].

A puzzle is that these quotes all seem to imply the belief, which seems widely held, is that genetic influences if such occurred, they should resemble a constant effect, invariant over countries, as if genes, their relative frequencies, and their estimates did not vary. One need only consider human height, a phenotypically genetically influenced sex difference variable, which varies in countries around the world both in the height of men and women and in the sizes of their mean differences [133].

Gene frequencies are known to often vary widely over different populations and countries due to migration factors, geography, climate, altitude, and mutations among other factors [134–137]. As the previous chapter's examples, analyses, and figures reveal, the relative size of $\hat{q}$ for the PISA data varies widely over different countries, both for math with $0.001 \leq \hat{q}_m \leq 0.476$ and for reading with $0.197 \leq \hat{q}_r \leq 0.614$.

As observed earlier, part of this variation seems plausibly attributed to geography and country history. And recall that The Czech Republic and Slovakia have among the largest PISA math q_m estimates, respectively, $\hat{q}_m = 0.302, 0.351$, from Table 5.3. These countries share a border and were earlier a single country. Norway and Sweden are another pair with a common border; their $\hat{q}$ for both reading and math will be considered below within another context. However, note here,

$\hat{q}_m = 0.026, 0.052$ for Norway and Sweden, respectively. Within each pair of these countries, the $\hat{q}_m$ seem similar, but between the pairs of countries the $\hat{q}_m$ are remarkable different.

It had been thought Europe was largely homogeneous in genetic variation. Recent palaeogenetical evidence clearly falsifies this belief and makes the variation in estimates of PISA q, over different countries, even more conceptually plausible. There were two genetically *distinct* groups in Europe around 30,000 years ago: one group living in France and Spain and the other group living in what is now The Czech Republic and in Italy [118, 119]. $\hat{q}_m = 0.050, 0.056$ PISA estimates for France and Spain, respectively. The Italian PISA estimate $\hat{q}_m = 0.144$, plus two additional Italian estimates $\hat{q}_m = 0.178(0.023), 0.237(0.028)$ with standard errors in parentheses, estimates from [60] appear to diverge from The Czech Republic PISA estimate $\hat{q}_m = 0.302$. But collectively the Czech Republic PISA and Italian q_m estimates are multiples larger of the France and Spain PISA $\hat{q}_m$. The $\hat{q}_r$ for these four countries seem more similar than do their $\hat{q}_m$ as Table 5.3 reveals. For France and Spain, respectively, $\hat{q}_r = 0.470, 0.464$. For The Czech Republic and Italy, $\hat{q}_r = 0.568, 0.417$, respectively.

An additional part of this variation, as already noted, in these parameter estimates is likely because they are different test translations, which may advantage boys and girls differently, depending on the language and culture. There is of course sampling variation in estimates, as noted earlier. What *is* nearly constant over countries are the inequalities in $\mathcal{S}$.

6.4 The Search for Biological Genetical Evidence

While $\mathcal{Y}$ models explicitly X-linked influences, other influences if they are plausibly viewed as being additive effects, both genetical and otherwise, can be represented through the location parameters μ_1 and μ_2. N can absorb variance changes. Consider the 1990 and 2017 eighth grade math means in Table 2.1. Both sexes increased 20 points over a 27 year interval. Component means $\hat{\mu}_1 = 262$ and 282 and $\hat{\mu}_2 = 407$ and 439, 1990, and 2017, respectively, reflecting these mean changes. The other parameter estimates remained similar. For example, $\hat{q} = 0.007$, and 0.006 for 1990 and 2017, respectively.

Genome wide association studies (GWAS) have become the most widely used approach for mapping genotype to phenotype associations [138]. These approaches, which may be viewed as a kind of data mining, can have serious difficulties because of linkage disequilibrium [139].

The core notion is that phenotypes are the results of thousands of minuscule genetical elements, SNPs (single-nucleotide polymorphisms), the outcomes of which additively combine, in a Mendelian matter, and are modelled as sums of random variables and are called polygenic scores. These scores are obtainable for individuals. Using polygenic scores for variables which may be considered proxies for an intelligence score, such as educational attainment, it has been claimed "... will bring the omnipotent variable of intelligence to all areas of the life sciences without the need to assess intelligence [140, p. 157]." For a very different perspective on this possibility, see Charney [141].

If the goal of understanding math and reading test score sex differences in task performance is seen as equivalent to the goal of coherently accounting of the inequalities of $\mathcal{S}$, which is the view here, then GWAS approaches, as currently constituted, appear unable to address the matter. There are a number of reasons for this conclusion. One is that GWAS requires huge sample sizes in the thousands or hundreds of thousands. Such a database for math and reading testing simply does not exist. More fundamental, however, is that the target traits for GWAS are *known* observable phenotypes. In $\mathcal{Y}$ the two phenotypes are unobserved latent distributions. GWAS approaches cannot address latent processes. To add a latent processes layer to the already complex GWAS framework would invariably increase outcome uncertainty which would seem to suggest the need for sample sizes perhaps unattainable for any variable of interest.

As stated before, at least for math, X-linked heritability is generally very small. So there is substantial variance unmodelled and unexplained. As just noted, the variable N or N_b for boys and N_g for girls reflects these contributions, some of which doubtlessly are polygene effects. There is no inconsistency here. A trait can have a major Mendelian influence as well as polygene influences. An unresolved issue in biology is where, along the continuous spectrum ranging from Mendelian genetics to complex polygene traits, particular phenotypes reside [142]. Whether current technology allows the biological identification of genes with small relative frequencies implied by $\mathcal{Y}$ seems unclear.

Genetical theory and its wide acceptance has been achieved historically through conceptual arguments and how these arguments "fit" with phenotypical data. It is difficult to find fault with $\mathcal{Y}$ on these grounds.

6.5 q as the Realization of a Random Variable Q

Because each individual V has been viewed throughout, as the unit of analysis, q may be viewed as random over different V. As Table 5.3 makes clear, $\hat{q}$ certainly varies widely, at the country level, for both reading and math. Within countries, there are doubtlessly subpopulations reflecting population flows over the ages, as well as the known stochastic behavior of genes [143]. Assuming q is a fixed unknown constant for any V is, as features of all models are, an approximation to reality. More realistically, $\hat{q}$ is a mean value of different values of q. This within V randomness, while not explicitly modeled, does not appear to jeopardize the core features of the model. The following argument hopefully makes this clear.

Let the random variable Q have realizations q and with continuous or discrete distribution function $G(q)$. Consider math for boys. Clearly, $P(B_b = \mu_2|q) = q$.

Then,

$$P(B_b = \mu_2) = \int P(B_b = \mu_2|q)dG(q) = \int qdG(q) = \mathrm{E}(Q).$$

So, estimates of q may be viewed as estimates of the mean of Q and similarly for girls.

6.6 Sex Differences in Distributional Tails

As has been noted above, a widely recognized empirical marker for sex differences particularly in math is observed differences in the test score distributional tails, with boys having larger math right tails than girls [11, 12, 144]. Often proxies for these differences, such as effect size or variance ratios, are of focus. The comparison of reading and math tail areas, both upper tail and lower tail, has also been observed: "The sex difference in mathematics was non-existent in the lower end of the performance distribution, but the sex difference in reading at the lower end was at its peak [122, p. 4]." The matter of right tail inequality is particularly concerning to Ceci and Williams [5]. They make reference to the "right tail" more than fifty times in their book.

That $\mathcal{Y}$ produces graphs which portray these tail area differences both for reading and for math is clear from the many figures displayed above. What is noted here is that with an additional distributional assumption, these differences follow from $\mathcal{Y}$.

Define

$$r(s) = \int_s^\infty f_b(y)dy \Big/ \int_s^\infty f_g(y)dy, -\infty < s < \infty.$$

If the component distributions of $f_b(y)$ and $f_g(y)$ are assumed to be normal, which is the assumption in the graphic displays when components appear, then $r(s)$ is strictly increasing as s increases (for the argument, see [104]). That is, the ratio of the upper tail areas not only favors boys over girls but also the ratio $r(s)$ will increase as, s, the smallest test score increases. American Mathematics Competition data [145] are consistent with the theory. A similar result holds for reading.

6.7 Two Additional Alternatives for *d*

In addition to the Hellinger distance, two other possible replacements for effect size d are suggested here. Neither require raw data. Their downsides are that they require specification of boys and girls test score probability distributions and computation with software. In the examples below, the component distributions are normal.

6.7.1 Girls Beat Boys

The spirit of this approach is by what proportion does one sex beat the other in test scores? Consider the probability $P(Y_b < Y_g)$, the proportion of girls' test scores which are greater than the boys' test scores. It is perhaps intuitively clear that if the random variables Y_b and Y_g shared the same continuous test score distribution, $P(Y_b < Y_g) = 1/2$. Then the departure of an observed proportion, $\hat{P}(Y_b < Y_g)$, from one-half expresses the separation of boys from girls. One might think pairs of boys and girls test scores would be required to assess the matter. However, this is not necessary as there is a general expression which is

$$P(Y_b < Y_g) = \int F_b(s) f_g(s) ds, -\infty < s < \infty,$$

where s is a test score. $F_b(s)$ is the lower tail cumulative probability distribution for boys and $f_g(s)$ the probability distribution (density) for girls. Both appear in Chap. 4. While the focus is on the distributions under $\mathcal{Y}$, the integral equation holds for all continuous probability distributions. Estimates $\widehat{F_b}(s)$ and $\hat{f_g}(s)$ are easily obtained by replacing their parameters with their estimates. Then a line or two of R code, using numerical integration, return $\hat{P}(Y_b < Y_g)$.

Using estimates obtained from the V associated with the U.S. 2003 PISA reading scores in Table 2.6 results in $\hat{P}(Y_b < Y_g) = 0.590$. Girls beat boys here.

6.7.2 The Overlap Coefficient OVL

OVL computes the amount of overlap between two distributions [146]. There are two versions: one for discrete distributions and one for continuous distributions.

$$OVL = \sum_y \min[f_b(y), f_g(y)],$$

which just sums the minimum height at each value of y. In a similar way for continuous data,

$$OVL = \int \min[f_b(y), f_g(y)] dy.$$

It is clear from these two definitions that if the distributions of boys and girls coincide, then $OVL = 1$, and if they share no support, that is, their distributions are disjoint, then $OVL = 0$.

OVL provides a useful way to portray how boys and girls are similar or different from each other with regard to their relative reading and math distributional overlap. Figures 6.1 and 6.2 display NAEP twelfth grade math and reading solutions.

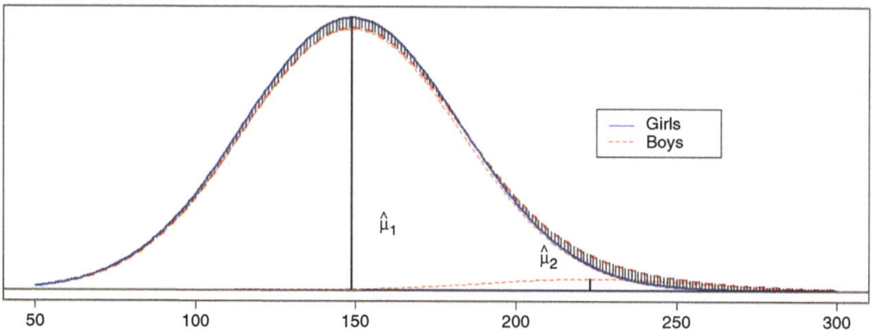

Fig. 6.1 NAEP 2019 Grade 12 math solution with V from Table 2.3. The unshaded area is the area of overlap

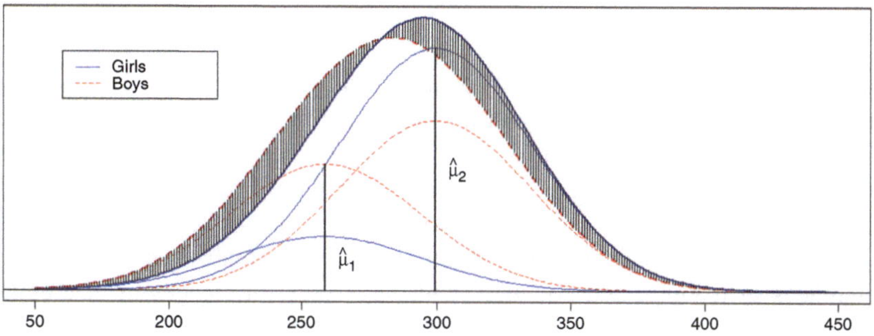

Fig. 6.2 NAEP 2015 Grade 12 reading solution with V from Table 2.4. The unshaded area is the area of overlap

Focus on $\hat{f}_g(y)$ the bold solid line and $\hat{f}_b(y)$ the bold dashed line. The white areas represent the overlap, while the shaded areas represent their corresponding distributional departures. The figures make clear there is much greater similarity in U.S. NAEP math scores at Grade 12 than in the NAEP reading scores at Grade 12. For math, $\widehat{OVL} = 0.971$, while for reading $\widehat{OVL} = 0.894$.

6.8 A PISA Reading and Math "Paradox"

This section addresses what is claimed to be a paradox. Addressing it is unrelated to matters pertaining to $\mathcal{Y}$, and thus it may be skipped if desired. But because the matter can be addressed with the data provided here and a resolution provided, the paradox is considered.

Figure 6.3 plots the difference scores girls' mean minus the boys' mean in reading, against the boys' mean minus the girls' mean in math, for all 41 countries with PISA data from Tables 2.5 and 2.6. $r = -0.589$. Marks [147] first reported such a

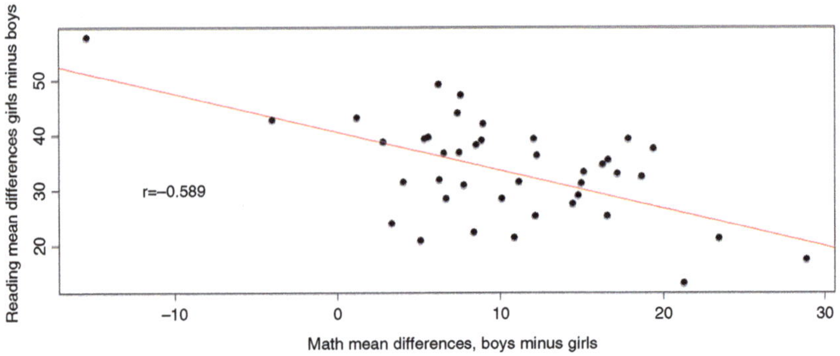

Fig. 6.3 Plot of 41 countries PISA reading mean differences, girls minus boys, against PISA math mean differences, boys minus girls. Data from Tables 2.5 and 2.6

relationship using PISA data from 25 countries. Stoet and Geary [122] provide four plots, their Figure 2, representing PISA data spanning a decade, with axes defined as in Fig. 6.3, which show $-0.78 \le r \le -0.60$. They regarded these negative correlations as very troubling: "…a hitherto unexplained paradoxical finding: The smaller the sex differences in mathematics, the larger the sex differences in reading (i.e., countries with a smaller sex difference in mathematics have a larger sex differences in reading, and countries with larger sex differences in mathematics have a smaller sex difference in reading). This inverse relation between the sex differences in mathematics and reading achievement poses a critical challenge for educators and policy makers who might wish to eliminate such differences … there are currently no countries that have successfully eliminated *both* the sex difference in mathematics… *and* the sex difference in reading… [122, p. 2, italics in original]."

In fact, the negative relationship can be the consequence of a simple obvious observation: Math skills are not required for reading test performance, but certainly some reading skills are necessary for some math test items. Girls hugely dominate boys' performance in reading. It has been noted [148] that girls' superior reading skill can lead them to opportunities where this skill is particularly advantageous. But it may not have been recognized that girls' reading skills would likely be advantageous as well for girls' understanding of at least some math test items, and thus their math and reading scores would be expected to be correlated. This correlation explains the paradox.

Assume that girls' reading and math scores are *positively* correlated. Then, *negative* correlations, as observed in, e.g., Fig. 6.3, fall out immediately as an expected empirical consequence. This result may seem counterintuitive.

To show this, define random variables B_{bm}, B_{gm}, B_{br}, and B_{gr}, where subscripts denote b for boys, g for girls, m for math, and r for reading. Thus, B_{gr} is a girl's reading score random variable. Let $\rho(\cdot)$ denote the correlation between pairs of random variables. Assume $\rho(B_{gm}, B_{gr}) > 0$, which is equivalent to the covariance $\text{cov}(B_{gm}, B_{gr}) > 0$. Other pairs of random variables are assumed independent of each other and thus are zero correlated.

Next, define

$$M = B_{bm} - B_{gm}$$

and

$$R = B_{gr} - B_{br}.$$

This pair of expressions is the probability model to evaluate. It is the sign of correlation between M and R, that is, $\rho(M, R)$, which is of concern. Because the sign of the covariance dictates the sign of the correlation, it is sufficient to consider the covariances, and without loss of generality, it may be assumed all random variables have zero mean.

$$\text{cov}(M, R) = \text{cov}(-B_{gm}, B_{gr}) = -\text{cov}(B_{gm}, B_{gr}) \Rightarrow \rho(M, R) < 0.$$

If for boys $\rho(B_{bm}, B_{br})$ were also assumed to be positive as well, as seems plausible, the same result would hold but drive $\rho(M, R)$ more negative. Thus, assuming that girls' math and reading scores are positively correlated is a sufficient condition to produce the negative M and R difference score correlation, and consequently the resulting empirical correlations, the negative rs, are simply realizations of what is expected.

Marks interpreted the correlation as having a causal thrust: "Policies that promote girls' educational performance decrease the gender gap in mathematics but also increase the gap in reading [147, p. 105]." If true, this conclusion is disturbing. Suppose a policy existed that could reduce the math gap by one-half. Then $\frac{1}{2}M = \frac{1}{2}(B_{bm} - B_{gm})$, which would shrink the expected mean difference in math by one-half. Under the model above, such a change has no influence on R, the reading gap, and in particular $\rho(\frac{1}{2}M, R) = \rho(M, R)$ leaving the correlation unchanged. Stoet and Geary [122] acknowledge they have no explanation for the paradox and claim further study is required. Given the above analysis, further study may not be needed.

6.9 Can *mdo* and *rdo* Be "Chance" Occurrences?

Could satisfying *rdo* or *mdo* simply be random chance events? The following focusses on math and *mdo*; the changes necessary for reading *rdo* should be apparent. Two very different answers must be given. As a first answer, assume boys' and girls' test scores are all independent and identically distributed, and based on random samples, and that their shared distribution is continuous. Then, $P(\bar{X}_b > \bar{X}_g) = P(S_b^2 > S_g^2) = 1/2$. Assuming in addition boys' and girls' test distributions are normal, then $P(\bar{X}_b > \bar{X}_g \cap S_b^2 > S_g^2) = 1/4$. The probability to consider if mdo is of focus is

$$p_m = P(\bar{X}_b > \bar{X}_g \cap S_b^2 > S_g^2 \cap S_b^2 - S_g^2 > \bar{X}_b - \bar{X}_g).$$

Under normality, $p_m < 1/4$ and is perhaps a crude upper bound. Otherwise, evaluating p_m would appear to require approximation by simulation. As an example, if test scores for both boys and girls followed a t distribution on $15 = df$, $p_m \approx 0.17$, with a sample size of 100 of each sex, a probability that appears roughly independent of sample size. Should $p_m \approx 1/4$, then a given V satisfying mdo could easily occur with sampling variation. However, given k independent V, the probability to consider is $1/4^k$, which becomes vanishing small as k grows. Consequently, a sampling variation argument is implausible given the large body of data reviewed above in Chap. 2.

This first answer just given applies to settings where it can be reasonably assumed that the elements of V were obtained from a random sample. For *none* of the large-scale national or international surveys, is this assumption appropriate, for reasons noted earlier, because the sampling and estimation procedures are far removed from a random sampling model. Thus, a second answer is required, but a definitive answer cannot be given. In the case of NAEP data, the consistency with which rdo and mdo hold over decades and with the knowledge that very large sample sizes are reflected in each sample estimated quantity will have to suffice. There are 66 NAEP V in Tables 2.1, 2.2, 2.3, and 2.4 for both reading and math. Among them, 58 satisfy either mdo or rdo. Assuming the V are independent of each other and assuming 1/4 would satisfy mdo or rdo by chance, the expected number is about 17. In the end, it is the pervasiveness of the empirical inequalities holding for children of various ages, over intervals spanning decades, in studies of varying size, globally and historically, for both reading and math that appears compelling and important. These empirical facts provide the ultimate justification for implementing $\mathcal{Y}$.

6.10 Model $\mathcal{Y}$ Dimensions and Fitting

The data of focus are two independent pairs of V $(\bar{x}_b, s_b)$ and $(\bar{x}_g, s_g)$ or four data points, while $\mathcal{Y}$ has four parameters, q, μ_1, μ_2, and σ. At first glance, one might think that the estimation and fitting procedures involving fitting four parameters to four data points results in a saturated model and consequently of little use. However, an examination of the model and estimation procedures shows that $\mathcal{Y}$ is a much more tightly constrained model than might first be thought, as has been stated earlier.

True, four parameters have been estimated in all the examples above. But as observed earlier, only three parameters are required to estimate the critical quantities and uniquely fix the graphical display properties: q, $\mu_2 - \mu_1$, and σ. Estimating μ_2 and μ_1 fixes the abscissa location of the display. Estimating only $\mu_2 - \mu_1$ changes nothing substantively in any of the above discussion. The graphs would then be unique within an abscissa translation. Furthermore, $\mathcal{Y}$ is a much more

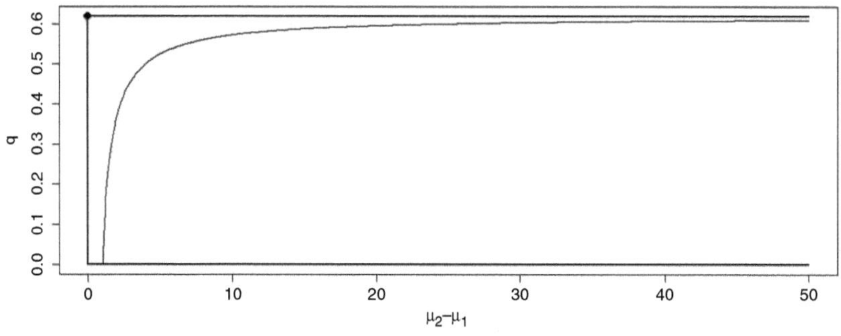

Fig. 6.4 Parameter space associated with $\mathcal{Y}$ inequalities. The rectangular space $0 < q < 0.618$ and $\mu_2 - \mu_1 > 0$ but is otherwise unbounded defines the space where inequalities (4.2) and (4.3) of Chap. 4 hold. The curved line denotes the space for inequality (4.4) to hold. These two parameters $\mu_2 - \mu_1 > 0$ and q generate the model inequalities

constrained model than counting the number of parameters reveals. Considering math, $\mathcal{Y}$ has three inequality constraints expressed in inequalities (4.2), (4.3), and (4.4) of Chap. 4, which correspond to the empirical inequalities of mo and mdo. In addition, an examination of these inequalities and their analytical arguments shows they are independent of σ, and thus the inequalities are forced by functions of just two parameters, $\mu_2 - \mu_1$ and q. Said in another way, the inequalities are forced by properties of B_b and B_g, while N_g and N_b play no role in generating $\mathcal{Y}$'s inequalities.

From a geometrical perspective, this means only a two-dimensional space is required to capture the parameter constraints, with two parameters q and $\mu_2 - \mu_1$ viewed as variables in this space. The space required to capture the model equivalent of mo is the rectangular graph shown in Fig. 6.4, open on the right side, because of the arbitrary upper bound $\mu_2 - \mu_1 \leq 50$ in the graph, but to capture mo only requires that $0 < q < 0.618$ and $\mu_1 < \mu_2$ or $0 < \mu_2 - \mu_1$.

To satisfy the model constraints corresponding to mdo, further constrains must be imposed: $\mu_2 - \mu_1 > 1$ and $q \leq [\sqrt{5 - 4/(\mu_2 - \mu_1)} - 1]/2 < 0.618$. The area below the curved line in Fig. 6.4 shows the corresponding model parameter space. Thus, Fig. 6.4 makes clear the analytical inequality properties of $\mathcal{Y}$ are determined by just two parameters. From a very different perspective, these results show just how readily falsifiable $\mathcal{Y}$ is. While the focus here has been on math, a similar development follows easily for reading.

6.11 $\mathcal{Y}$ and the Global Gender Gap Index

Yearly, the World Economic Forum releases an index of gender equality for each of about 150 different countries. Called the Global Gender Gap Index, or here GGGI, is a zero to one bounded scalar index, with one presumably denoting equality. It is a composite of four assessed domains for equality: economic participation and opportunities, educational attainment, health and survival, and political empowerment. GGGI is billed as a measure of "gender equality," which "assesses countries on how well they are dividing their resources and opportunities among their male and female populations, regardless of the overall levels of these resources and opportunities [149]." Any departure of the GGGI from one *by design* indexes only women's disadvantage. The measure cannot reflect any disadvantage for boys or men. Intuitively, this fact seems to violate the very premise of a symmetrical equality relation which the idea of "gender equality" seems to imply. The GGGI index for 2022 for the OECD PISA countries is given in Table 5.4, column four [150]. These values generally change modestly from year to year.

It is interesting to consider the range of GGGI values from the perspective of $\mathcal{Y}$. The assumption in doing so is that country-wide indices of sex differences in testing for both math and reading, as indexed by PISA scores, have wider implications. Although assessing children with tests is usually motivated by efforts to assess educational progress or use for selection purposes, it is arguably the case tests might be taken as a proxy index portending, in perhaps difficult ways to model or quantify, sex differences in behaviors reflected in various domains of activity long after the tests are taken, perhaps indicating individual life trajectories in a country. Furthermore, because girls show some marginal disadvantage in math scores in almost all OECD countries, such influences should modestly suppress GGGI scores. That is because they would likely increase disparities in domains that would contribute to that country's index, thus lowering the GGGI value for the country. However, girls show a huge advantage in all OECD countries on PISA reading tests, and thus, reading score indices should be positively associated with GGGI scores. It is difficult to specify any *waking* activity in modern culture which is independent, or at least uncorrelated, with the ability to read. It is possible to be more quantitatively precise. In doing so, all data employed in this section are in Tables 5.3 and 5.4.

Consider first math. To remind the reader, letting q_m denote q for math, the upper component latent math distribution was weighted q_m for boys and q_m^2 for girls, and the component weights were the only features that marked their distributions as different. Recall $q_m - q_m^2 > 0$ for $0 < q_m < 1$. The difference $q_m - q_m^2$ is smallest for q_m small, and this difference strictly increases in q_m for $0 < q_m \leq 1/2$. This leads to the prediction that as the difference $q_m - q_m^2$ increases, signaling wider sex disparities in various domains for which math performance has relevance, the GGGI should modestly decrease. There are 30 countries in Tables 5.3 and 5.4 where pairs of these variables are available. Using notation that should be intuitively clear, the corresponding correlation is $r(\hat{q}_m - \hat{q}_m^2, GGGI) = -0.313(0.165)$ with standard error in parenthesis. The corresponding scatter plot appears in Fig. 6.5.

Consider reading: the reasoning is identical to that for math, with q_r denoting the reading q. The girls' latent higher scoring reading component weight is $1 - q_r^2$, which is larger than the boys' component weight of $1 - q_r$. Thus, $(1 - q_r^2) - (1 - q_r) = q_r - q_r^2$, so precisely the same correlational structure of math and GGGI is of focus for reading except that a positive correlation is expected. Retaining the same

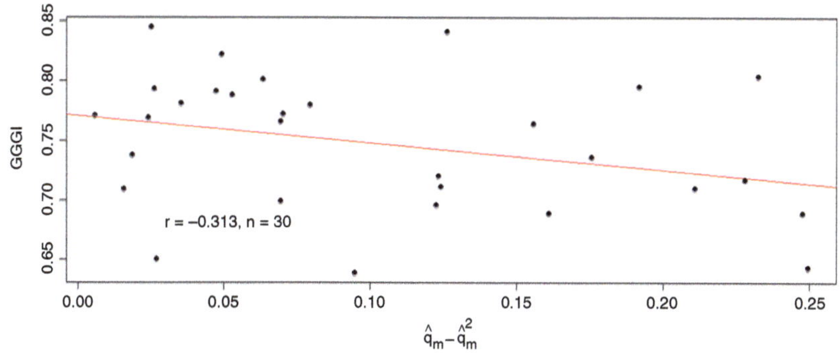

Fig. 6.5 Scatter plot of GGGI against $\hat{q}_m - \hat{q}_m^2$

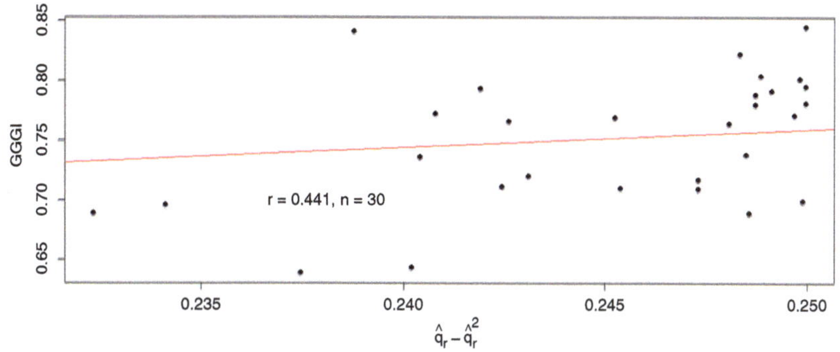

Fig. 6.6 Scatter plot of GGGI against $\hat{q}_r - \hat{q}_r^2$ for 29 countries. Japan with coordinates (0.158, 0.650) is not shown. If Japan were excluded, $r = 0.456$ for 29 countries

30 countries as before, $r(\hat{q}_r - \hat{q}_r^2, GGGI) = 0.441(0.147)$ with standard error in parenthesis. The corresponding scatter plot appears in Fig. 6.6, while $r(\hat{q}_m - \hat{q}_m^2, \hat{q}_r - \hat{q}_r^2) = 0.112$.

More broadly, these findings seem noteworthy. For one, they increase the plausibility of the wide variability of $\hat{q}$ for reading and math among countries, and for another, would seem to allow for $\mathcal{Y}$ to be viewed as having saliency within a wider context. The predictions are model-based, and the estimated proportion of the variance in the GGGI accounted for by the two PISA tests is 0.327 (please see Appendix A.5 for clarification).

The above exposition views GGGI indices, in part at least, as a *consequence* of the same factors, under $\mathcal{Y}$, that produce sex differences in reading and math test scores. Other perspectives view the causal suggestion as going in the opposite direction: countries with high GGGI, or other similar indices of country-wide social equality, are viewed as incubators for, if not causal agents for reducing sex differences in math [19]. Furthermore, at the same time, as the math gap for girls is presumably under reduction because of social forces, the same social forces are *increasing* the reading gap advantage for girls [151]. There is, apparently, no safe harbor for boys with their substantial mean reading gap.

An article's headline summary is "Analysis of PISA results suggests that the gender gap in *math* scores *disappears* in countries with a more gender-equal culture [151, p. 1164, italics added]." Now replace the first and second italicized words with, respectively, *reading* and *increases.* Doing so one has an alternative description of their findings.

The article's goal is to convince the reader that "... in countries with a higher GGI index (here GGGI), girls close the gender gap by becoming both better in math and reading, not by closing the math gap alone [151, p. 1165]." And they contend that "In more gender-equal countries, such as Norway and Sweden, the math gender gap disappears [151, p. 1164]." The authors repeatedly state that in more gender-equal countries the math gender-gap "disappears."

While the implied causal linkage between countries with high GGGI and girls' math achievement already appears suspect [152], there is another difficulty: the claim the gap disappears in high GGGI countries is misleading hyperbole. The gender gap does not disappear, nor are the Norway and Sweden math differences especially small. For both countries, $6 < \bar{x}_b - \bar{x}_g < 7$. For 12 of the 37 countries with both GGGI and PISA scores, the math differences are less than 7, and for two of these countries the differences are negative, as the data in Table 2.5 reveal. It is notable in this context that the U.S. math gap is 6.25, less than Sweden's gap of 6.53. This U.S. math gap has not been claimed, in the U.S.A. at least, to have "disappeared."

Norway and Sweden were featured in the authors' chart [151, p. 1164] because in 2006, their GGGI values were, along with Finland, the highest. Then, Norway's GGGI was 0.799 and for Sweden 0.813 [149]. In Table 5.4, the 2022 values show Norway has the third largest among 37 countries with GGGI of 0.845, and Swedens' 0.822 is the fifth largest.

The authors, as well as here, apparently employ the 2003 PISA cycle data. Whether the source files are identical, however, cannot be determined. For 37 countries with GGGI values and PISA scores, for math, $r(\bar{x}_b - \bar{x}_g, GGGI) = -0.426$, so smaller math disparities are associated with higher GGGI.

The problem with the authors' interpretation arises when reading is considered. If countries with equitable resource distribution are credited with reducing math disparities, would not it be plausible to expect reading disparities would be reduced as well? This is most certainly not the case. For PISA reading differences, $r(\bar{x}_g - \bar{x}_b, GGGI) = 0.494$ signaling that as GGGI increases, so does the reading gap. The authors claim, as they must, and as implausible as it would seem, that a country's gender equality *increases* reading disparities. This does not imply of course that *all* of the $\bar{x}_g - \bar{x}_b > 0$ of the PISA reading differences are attributable to the presumed influence of a country's gender equality. For their two featured countries, Norway and Sweden, the reading scores hugely favor girls.

For Norway, the difference in means is 49.2, the second largest among 41 countries in Table 2.6; Sweden's difference is 36.75 well above the median of 33.34. These differences are many times the size of their math differences. These mean differences favoring girls in reading would seem to well exceed the sizes of socially or environmentally based influences for nearly *any* variable of interest. So, what is there about a country's gender equality that works dramatically differently on math to *decrease* disparities than it does on reading to *increase* disparities? Is it to be claimed that social equality forces only lift girls' scores? The issue is not addressed.

The expected math mean test score difference between boys and girls under $\mathcal{Y}$ is

$$\mathrm{E}(Y_b - Y_g) = q(1-q)(\mu_2 - \mu_1) > 0, 0 < q < 1, \mu_1 < \mu_2,$$

showing the math gap increases as $q \to 1/2$ and it approaches zero as $q \to 0$. It is also largest for a fixed $\mu_2 - \mu_1 > 0$ when $q = 1/2$. (Replace the left side with $\mathrm{E}(Y_g - Y_b)$ for reading.)

The $\mathcal{Y}$ interpretation for reading and math for Sweden and Norway is quite different of course. First note that for both countries $\widehat{V}$ for both reading and math are nearly identical with their V. $\hat{q}_m$ is small for both countries, and that is why the math mean sex differences are small. For Norway, $\hat{q}_m = 0.026$ and for Sweden $\hat{q}_m = 0.052$, the seventh and thirteen smallest values among those in Table 5.3. For reading, for Sweden $\hat{q}_r = 0.541$, and for Norway $\hat{q}_r = 0.506$, the fifth and eighth largest values in Table 5.3. Because the $\hat{q}_r$ are large, the reading mean difference is large. The rough similarity in these two countries' q estimates for both reading and math would seem to be best understood, as suggested before, by their geography, a fact not mentioned in the article of focus. The two countries share a 1630 kilometer border and thus are thought to share similar gene pools [120].

Another application of GGGI has led to a spectacular failure. It was expected there would be a positive correlation between women's participation in college level math focused curricula among different countries and their GGGI index. Instead, a strikingly negative correlation, $r = -0.47$, appeared, a finding called a paradox by Stoet and Geary [153]. This is the second such correlational finding so labelled by them as a paradox. The first "paradox" was discussed above in Sect. 6.8.

The most common explanation for such findings continues to be gender stereotyping. Subsequently, a gender stereotype variable, GMS, yielded $r(GMS, GGGI) = 0.291$ for OECD countries [154, p. 30, Table S4A], the most suitable comparison for the data available here. For a larger sample of countries, $r(GMS, GGGI) = 0.434$ [155, Table 1]. Thus, GMS accounts for about 9% or at most about 19% of the variance of GGGI. Using both math and reading PISA tests, $\mathcal{Y}$ accounts for nearly one-third of the GGGI variance, 32.7% and given above, well more than does GMS.

While such correlations may be of interest, the spirit of a core global issue seems best captured by observations of Ceci and Williams [5, p. 168] And discussed earlier: why is the male to female ratio of computer scientists in The Czech Republic more than six, while in the U.S.A. that ratio is about two? To the extent to which PISA math scores address the matter and to briefly return to that discussion here, $\mathcal{Y}$ provides at least part of the answer. Figure 6.7 shows the estimated upper tail distribution functions under $\mathcal{Y}$ for both the U.S.A. and The Czech Republic assuming component normality. The upper tail sex differences are

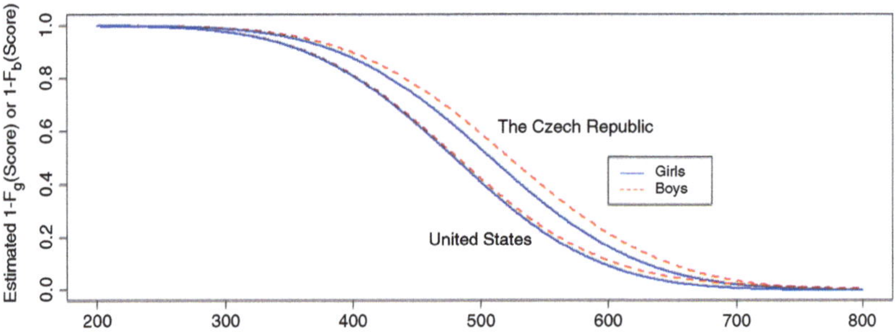

Fig. 6.7 Estimated distribution function upper tails for PISA math for boys and girls, The Czech Republic and the United States

far more pronounced in The Czech Republic than in the U.S.A., largely because $\hat{q}_m = 0.306$ and 0.025 for The Czech Republic and U.S.A., respectively, and as noted earlier. For both countries, the $\widehat{V}$ match their V reported in Table 2.5.

The GGGI indices employed in the above analyses are from 2022, while the PISA data are from the 2003 assessment cycle. Thus, nearly two decades separates the assessment times of the two variables of focus. This fact would seem to suggest that the durability of the findings is to be expected.

Finally, please keep in mind that *none* of the references in this section which attempt to address the mean gender gap in math consider variance differences, the largest of the sex differences in both math and reading testing. To repeat yet again, any coherent explanation of sex differences must jointly address the variance differences as well as the mean differences. Only $\mathcal{Y}$ has, so far, achieved that status.

6.12 The Misleading Language and Images of Sex Differences

Both the language psychologists have used to refer to sex differences, and the graphical images drawn to portray such differences have been misleading.

Consider language first. Words can shape beliefs and perceptions. Perhaps no two words have been used more often to characterize sex differences, certainly with respect to math and secondarily with respect to reading (as well as many other domains of focus) than "gender gap." Search with the words "gender gap" in any browser and millions of hits are revealed. Gender gap appears in the titles of several books; it appears in three of fifteen chapter titles in a single book addressing math sex differences [79] and 128 times in single book [5]. Gender gap appears rarely explicitly defined, but it seems clear that it is taken to mean sample mean test score differences at least where math and reading are of focus. The popularity of the two words being so, gender gap would seem to fail to satisfy a "real" definition, meaning to convey the "essential nature" or "essential attributes" of some entity [75, p. 93].

Certainly, in math testing, $\bar{x}_b - \bar{x}_g > 0$ typically. So considering gender gap as equivalent to boys' and girls' mean math test score difference is not wrong.

However, once it is recognized how widely the inequality *mdo* holds and when it is realized how much larger $s_b^2 - s_g^2$ is than $\bar{x}_b - \bar{x}_g$ for math, any "essential nature" scalar characterizing sex differences in math and reading should be the variance difference. The median of the 41 ratios $(s_b^2 - s_g^2)/|\bar{x}_b - \bar{x}_g|$ for PISA math scores of Table 2.5 is 111. For PISA reading scores, Table 2.6, the median of the ratio is 46. Is it unreasonable to suggest that for many years the focus has been on the mean gender gap when it should be on the variance gender gap?

The figures or graphs of distributions intended to portray sex differences in math are misleading. Invariably, portrayed are equal variance but shifted normal distributions. This is certainly an empirically wrong visual image, and it is conceptually misleading as well.

6.13 Coda

In the executive summary of *Why So Few?* a book that concerns why there are few women in math and related fields, the authors write "While biological gender differences, yet to be well understood, may play a role, they clearly are not the whole story [156, p. xiv]." Nothing written in these chapters contradicts the spirit of this statement. What has been shown, however, is that virtually all of the reading and math test-based sex differences displayed by children in observational settings, especially those of $\mathcal{S}$, can be explained by a simple model.

View the foregoing effort as an attempt to advance understanding of the biological basis of the differences expressed in the above quote. In the process, the effort has hopefully illuminated the far larger mean difference favoring girls in reading that has been mostly ignored. It is literacy, not math, that is the far larger and more important skill for children to acquire.

It would appear time to focus attention on the multitude of those sex differences which are most likely under some form of environmental or societal control and not mentioned above.

Appendix A
Arguments, Estimation, and R Code

A.1 The Distribution of Y

The unconditional distribution of $Y = B + N$.

Set $P(B = \mu_k) = \pi_k, \pi_1 + \pi_2 = 1, 0 < \pi_k < 1, k = 1, 2$. The cumulative distribution function of Y is $F(y) = P(Y \le y) = \sum_{k=1}^{2} P(Y \le y, B = \mu_k) = \sum_{k=1}^{2} P(Y \le y|B = \mu_k)P(B = \mu_k)$. Write $P(Y \le y|B = \mu_k) = F_k(y)$, and then $F(y) = P(Y \le y) = \pi_1 F_1(y) + \pi_2 F_2(y)$. If $f(y)$ is either a probability mass function or a density function, then $f(y) = \pi_1 f_1(y) + \pi_2 f_2(y)$. The distributions for reading and math, for boys and girls, are then easily specified.

A.2 Inequality Arguments

The Y mean, variance, and inequality arguments for math:

Conditions: $\mu_1 < \mu_2, 0 < q < 1$, so $q^2 < q$ for all q.

$$\mathrm{E}(Y_b) = \mu_b = (1 - q)\mu_1 + q\mu_2 \tag{A.1}$$

$$\mathrm{E}(Y_g) = \mu_g = (1 - q^2)\mu_1 + q^2\mu_2. \tag{A.2}$$

From (A.1) and (A.2),

$$\mu_b > \mu_g \tag{A.3}$$

$$\mathrm{var}(Y_b) = \sigma_b^2 = (\mu_2 - \mu_1)^2 q(1 - q) + \sigma^2 \tag{A.4}$$

$$\mathrm{var}(Y_g) = \sigma_g^2 = (\mu_2 - \mu_1)^2 q^2(1 - q^2) + \sigma^2. \tag{A.5}$$

H. Thomas, *Sex Differences in Reading and Math Test Scores of Children*,
Monographs in the Psychology of Education,
https://doi.org/10.1007/978-3-031-41272-1

From (A.4) and (A.5),

$$\sigma_b^2 > \sigma_g^2 \iff 0 > q(1+q) - 1 \iff q < .618 = \frac{\sqrt{5}-1}{2}. \tag{A.6}$$

From (A.1), (A.2), (A.4), and (A.5) with $\mu_2 - \mu_1 = \mu_d > 0$. If

$$L = \{\mu_d = \mu_2 - \mu_1 > 1 \;\&\; 0 < q < ([5 - 4/\mu_d]^{1/2} - 1)/2 < .618\} \tag{A.7}$$

and L in (A.7) holds, then

$$\sigma_b^2 - \sigma_g^2 > \mu_b - \mu_g. \tag{A.8}$$

The argument for (A.8):

$$\sigma_b^2 - \sigma_g^2 = q(1-q)\mu_d^2[1 - q(1+q)] \tag{A.9}$$

$$\mu_b - \mu_g = q(1-q)\mu_d \tag{A.10}$$

$$\begin{aligned}\sigma_b^2 - \sigma_g^2 > \mu_b - \mu_g &\iff \mu_d[1 - q(1+q)] > 1 \\ &\iff -\mu_d q^2 - \mu_d q + \mu_d - 1 > 0\end{aligned} \tag{A.11}$$

$$q = \frac{\sqrt{5 - 4/\mu_d} - 1}{2}. \tag{A.12}$$

Inspection of (A.12) reveals that for $q > 0$ it must be that $\mu_d > 1$; if $\mu_d = \infty$, then $q = \frac{\sqrt{5}-1}{2} = .618$. Thus, for (A.8) to hold, L must hold.

A similar development follows for reading.

A.3 Estimation Algorithm

The moment estimation algorithm for math, given *mo*:

Step 1: Execute (A.13) and (A.14):

$$\omega = \frac{(\bar{x}_b - \bar{x}_g)^2}{s_b^2 - s_g^2} = \frac{(\mu_b - \mu_g)^2}{\sigma_b^2 - \sigma_g^2} = \frac{q(1-q)}{1 - q(1+q)} \tag{A.13}$$

$$\hat{q} = \frac{1 + \omega - \sqrt{5\omega^2 - 2\omega + 1}}{2(1-\omega)} \tag{A.14}$$

$$\bar{x}_b - \bar{x}_g = \mu_b - \mu_g = (\mu_2 - \mu_1)q(1-q) \tag{A.15}$$

$$s_b^2 - s_g^2 = \sigma_b^2 - \sigma_g^2 = (\mu_2 - \mu_1)^2 q(1-q)[1 - q(1+q)] \tag{A.16}$$

$$\bar{x}_b = \mu_b = (1-q)\mu_1 + q\mu_2 \tag{A.17}$$

$$\bar{x}_g = \mu_g = (1-q^2)\mu_1 + q^2\mu_2 \tag{A.18}$$

$$s_b^2 = \sigma^2 + q(1-q)(\mu_2 - \mu_1)^2 \tag{A.19}$$

$$s_g^2 = \sigma^2 + q^2(1-q^2)(\mu_2 - \mu_1)^2. \tag{A.20}$$

Step 2: Estimate $\mu_d = \mu_2 - \mu_1$ using (A.14) and (A.16):

$$\hat{\mu}_d = (\widehat{\mu_2 - \mu_1}) = \sqrt{(s_b^2 - s_g^2)/\hat{q}(1-\hat{q})[1 - \hat{q}(1+\hat{q})]}. \tag{A.21}$$

Using (A.14) and (A.15),

$$\hat{\mu}_d = (\widehat{\mu_2 - \mu_1}) = (\bar{x}_b - \bar{x}_g)/\hat{q}(1-\hat{q}). \tag{A.22}$$

(A.22) is used in the algorithm.
Step 3: Estimate σ^2 using (A.19) and (A.20).

$$\dot{\sigma}^2 = s_b^2 - \hat{\mu}_d^2\hat{q}(1-\hat{q}) \tag{A.23}$$

and

$$\dot{\sigma}^2 = s_g^2 - \hat{\mu}_d^2\hat{q}^2(1-\hat{q}^2). \tag{A.24}$$

The two $\dot{\sigma}^2$ are averaged and set equal to $\hat{\sigma}^2$ if they are positive. Estimates can be negative, so-called Heywood cases in which case estimation fails.

Three parameters are estimated above, μ_d, q, and σ^2, so the estimation is complete save for translations of $\hat{f}_b(y)$ and $\hat{f}_g(y)$ on the real line. However, μ_k can be estimated to uniquely fix their locations.

Step 4: Estimate μ_k:

$$\hat{\mu}_1 = \frac{\bar{x}_g - \hat{q}\bar{x}_b}{1-\hat{q}} \tag{A.25}$$

$$\hat{\mu}_2 = \frac{(1+\hat{q})\bar{x}_b - \bar{x}_g}{\hat{q}}. \tag{A.26}$$

The following provides the argument for (A.25) and (A.26).

$$\begin{pmatrix} a & b \\ c & d \end{pmatrix}^{-1} = \frac{1}{(ad-bc)} \begin{pmatrix} d & -b \\ -c & a \end{pmatrix}. \tag{A.27}$$

Rewriting (A.17) and (A.18),

$$\begin{pmatrix} \bar{x}_b \\ \bar{x}_g \end{pmatrix} = \begin{pmatrix} 1-\hat{q} & \hat{q} \\ 1-\hat{q}^2 & \hat{q}^2 \end{pmatrix} \begin{pmatrix} \hat{\mu}_1 \\ \hat{\mu}_2 \end{pmatrix}. \tag{A.28}$$

Using (A.27),

$$\begin{pmatrix} 1-\hat{q} & \hat{q} \\ 1-\hat{q}^2 & \hat{q}^2 \end{pmatrix}^{-1} = \frac{1}{\hat{q}(\hat{q}-1)} \begin{pmatrix} \hat{q}^2 & -\hat{q} \\ \hat{q}^2-1 & 1-\hat{q} \end{pmatrix}. \tag{A.29}$$

Using (A.28) and (A.29),

$$\begin{pmatrix} \hat{\mu}_1 \\ \hat{\mu}_2 \end{pmatrix} = \frac{1}{\hat{q}(\hat{q}-1)} \begin{pmatrix} \hat{q}^2 & -\hat{q} \\ \hat{q}^2-1 & 1-\hat{q} \end{pmatrix} \begin{pmatrix} \bar{x}_b \\ \bar{x}_g \end{pmatrix} \tag{A.30}$$

giving (A.25) and (A.26). Note (A.26) minus (A.25) equals (A.22). The changes required for estimates of reading V should be clear.

A.4 R Function `mathgap`

Math estimation algorithm in R. Required is vector v lower case with four or six elements satisfying *mo*.

```
mathgap<-function(){
  mb<-v[1];mg<-v[2];vb<-v[3]^2;vg<-v[4]^2
  nv<-c("q","q^2","md","m1","m2","v(N)","vxb","vxg","h^2_b",
        "h^2_g","tvb","tvg")
  if(length(v)==4){
    d<-((mb-mg)^2)/(vb-vg)
    estq<-((1+d)-sqrt(5*d^2-2*d+1))/(2*(1-d))
    m1<-(v[2]-estq*v[1])/(1-estq)
    m2<-((1+estq)*v[1]-v[2])/estq
    md<-m2-m1
    vxlb<-md^2*estq*(1-estq);vxlg<-md^2*(estq^2)*(1-estq^2)
    vs<-c(vb-md^2*estq*(1-estq),vg-md^2*estq^2*(1-estq^2))
    if(sum(vs>0)==2)vstuff<-mean(vs)else
    {print("Heywood");vstuff<-max(vs)}
    gv<<-pv<-c(estq,estq^2,md,m1,m2,vstuff,vxlb,vxlg,
               vxlb/(vxlb+vstuff),vxlg/(vxlg+vstuff),
               vstuff+vxlb,vstuff+vxlg)
    names(pv)<-nv
    pv<-round(pv,3)
```

```
    return(pv)
  }
  if(length(v)==6){
    nb<-v[5];ng<-v[6]
    d<-((mb-mg)^2-(vb/nb+vg/ng))/(vb-vg)
    if(d<0) d<-((mb-mg)^2)/(vb-vg)
    estq<-((1+d)-sqrt(5*d^2-2*d+1))/(2*(1-d))
    m1<-(v[2]-estq*v[1])/(1-estq)
    m2<-((1+estq)*v[1]-v[2])/estq
    md<-m2-m1
    vxlb<-md^2*estq*(1-estq);vxlg<-md^2*(estq^2)*(1-estq^2)
    vs<-c(vb-md^2*estq*(1-estq),vg-md^2*estq^2*(1-estq^2))
    if(sum(vs>0)==2){vstuff<-(vs[1]*nb+vs[2]*ng)/(nb+ng)} else
    {print("Heywood");vstuff<-max(vs)}
    gv<<-pv<-c(estq,estq^2,md,m1,m2,vstuff,vxlb,vxlg,
               vxlb/(vxlb+vstuff),vxlg/(vxlg+vstuff),
               vstuff+vxlb,vstuff+vxlg)
  }
  names(pv)<-nv
  pv<-round(pv,3)
  return(pv)
  }
```

A.5 Conditional r Variance

The proportion of variance of x given y and z.

Suppose there are three variables, x, y, and z, with r_{xy} denoting the sample correlation coefficient between x and y and similarly r_{xz} and r_{yz}. Desired is the estimated proportion of the variance of x accounted for by y and z. The expression is

$$\frac{1}{1-r_{yz}^2}(r_{xy}^2 + r_{xz}^2 - 2r_{xy}r_{xz}r_{yz}).$$

The expression is distribution free, but the linearity of the corresponding regressions is assumed. For application here, set $x = GGGI$, $y = \hat{q}_m - \hat{q}_m^2$, and $z = \hat{q}_r - \hat{q}_r^2$.

References

1. Rice, J. M. (1897). The Futility of the spelling grind II. *The Forum, 34*, 409–419.
2. Rice, J. M. (1902). Educational research: A test in arithmetic. *The Forum, 34*, 281–297.
3. Stone, C. W. (1908). *Arithmetical abilities and some factors determining them*. New York: Teachers College, Columbia University. Republished by BiblioLife, LLC, Charleston, SC, in 2021.
4. Gray, W. S. (1917). *Studies of elementary-school reading through standardized tests*. Chicago: University of Chicago Press.
5. Ceci, S. J., & Williams, W. M. (2010). *The mathematics of sex: How biology and society conspire to limit talented women and girls*. New York: Oxford University Press. https://doi.org/10.1037/a0014412
6. Murray, C. (2020). *Human diversity: The biology of gender, race, and class*. New York: Twelve.
7. Lakin, J. M. (2013). Sex differences in reasoning abilities: Surprising evidence that male-female ratios in the tails of quantitative reasoning distribution have increased. *Intelligence, 41*, 263–274. https://doi.org/10.1016/j.intell.2013.04.004
8. Hyde, J. S., Fennema, E., & Lamon, S. J. (1990). Gender differences in mathematics performance: A meta-analysis. *Psychological Bulletin, 107*, 139–155. https://doi.org/10.1037/0033-2909.107.2.139
9. Hyde, J. S., Lindberg, S. M., Linn, M. C., Ellis, A. B., & Williams, C. C. (2008). Gender similarities characterize math performance. *Science, 321*, 494–495. https://doi.org/10.1126/science.1160364
10. Lindberg, S. M., Hyde, J. S., Petersen, J. L., & Linn, M. C. (2010). New trends in mathematics performance: A meta-analysis. *Psychological Bulletin, 136*(6), 1123–1135. https://doi.org/10.1037/a0021276
11. Baye, A., & Monseur, C. (2016). Gender differences in variability and extreme scores in international context. *Large-Scale Assessments in Education, 4*, 3–16. https://doi.org/10.1186/s40536-015-0015-x
12. Halpern, D. F., Benbow, C. P., Geary, D. C., Gur, R. C., Hyde, J. S., & Gernsbacher, M. A. (2007). The science of sex differences in science and mathematics. *Psychological Science in the Public Interest, 8*, 1–51. https://doi.org/10.1111/j.1529-1006.2007.00032.x
13. Hedges, L. V., & Nowell, A. (1995). Sex differences in mental scores, variability, and numbers of high-scoring individuals. *Science, 269*, 41–45. https://doi.org/10.1126/science.7604277
14. Lynn, R., & Mikk, J. (2009). Sex differences in reading achievement. *TRAMES. A Journal of the Humanities and Social Sciences, 13*(63/58), 1, 3–13.

H. Thomas, *Sex Differences in Reading and Math Test Scores of Children*, Monographs in the Psychology of Education, https://doi.org/10.1007/978-3-031-41272-1

15. Hyde, J. S., Bigler, R. S., Joel, D., Tate, C. C., & van Andrews, S. M. (2019). The future of sex and gender in psychology: Five challenges to the gender binary. *American Psychologist, 74*, 171–193. https://doi.org/10.1037/amp0000307
16. Tversky, A., & Kahneman, D. (1974). Judgment under uncertainty: Heuristics and biases. *Science, 185*, 1124–1131. https://doi.org/10.1126/science.185.4157.1124
17. Feingold, A. (1988). Cognitive gender differences are disappearing. *American Psychologist, 43*(2), 95–103. https://doi.org/10.1037/0003-066X.43.2.95
18. Miller, D. I., & Halpern, D. F. (2014). The new science of cognitive sex differences. *Trends in Cognitive Sciences, 18*(1), 37–45. https://doi.org/10.1016/j.tics.2013.10.011
19. Breda, T., Jouini, E., Napp, C., & Thebault, G. (2018). Society inequalities amplify gender gaps in math. *Science, 359*, 1219–1220. https://doi.org/10.1126/science.aar2307
20. Casey, B., & Ganley, C. M. (2021). An examination of gender differences in spatial skills and math attitudes in relation to mathematics success: A bio-psycho-social model. *Developmental Review, 60*, 100963. https://doi.org/10.1016/j.dr.2021.100963
21. Staddon, J. (2022). *Science in an age of unreason*. Washington, DC: Regnery Gateway.
22. Coyne, J. A., & Krylov, A. L. (2023). The 'hurtful' idea of scientific merit. *The Wall Street Journal*, A17.
23. Eagly, A. H., & Revelle, W. (2022). Understanding the magnitude of psychological differences between women and men requires seeing the forest and the trees. *Perspectives on Psychological Science, 17*(5), 1339–1358. https://doi.org/10.1177/17456916211046006
24. Pearl, J., & Mackenzie, D. (2018). *The book of why*. New York: Basic Books.
25. Hyde, J. S. (2014). Gender similarities and differences. *Annual Review of Psychology, 65*, 373–398. https://doi.org/10.1146/annurev-psych-010213-115057
26. Aitkin, M., & Aitkin, I. (2011). *Statistical modeling of the national assessment of educational progress*. Springer: New York. https://doi.org/10.1007/978-1-4419-9937-5
27. Efron, B., & Tibshirani, R. J. (1993). *An introduction to the bootstrap*. New York: Chapman & Hall. https://doi.org/10.1007/978-1-4899-4541-9
28. Feingold, A. (1992). Sex differences in variability in intellectual abilities: A new look at an old controversy. *Review of Educational Research, 62*, 61–84. https://doi.org/10.3102/00346543062001061
29. Burt, S. A., & Johnson, W. (2022). Joint consideration of means and variances might change the understanding of etiology. *Perspectives on Psychological Science, 18*(2), 416–427. https://doi.org/10.1177/17456916221096122
30. NDE. (2022). The Nation's Report Card. https://www.nationsreportcard.gov/ndecore/xplore/NDE
31. Hyde, J. S., Lindberg, S. M., Linn, M. C., Ellis, A. B., & Williams, C. C. (2008). Supporting Online Material for Gender similarities characterize math performance. *Science, 321*, 494–495. https://doi.org/10.1126/Science.1160364
32. Hyde, J. S., & Linn, M. C. (2006). Gender similarities in mathematics and science. *Science, 314*, 599–600. https://doi.org/10.1126/science.1132154
33. Hyde, J. S., & Mertz, J. E. (2009). Gender, culture, and mathematics performance. *Proceedings the National Academy of Sciences, 106*, 8801–8807. https://doi.org/10.1073/pnas.0901265106
34. Kagan, J. (2012). *Psychology's ghosts: The crisis in the profession and the way back*. New Haven: Yale.
35. Nosek, B. A., Alter, G., Banks, G. C., Borsboom, D., Bowman, S. D., Breckler, S. J., et al. (2015). Promoting an open research culture. *Science, 348*(6242), 1422–1425. https://doi.org/10.1126/science.aab2374
36. Mullis, I. V. S. (2019). *White Paper on 50 Years of NAEP Use: Where NAEP Has Been and Where It Should Go Next*. Commissioned by the NAEP Validity Studies (NVS) Panel.
37. Jones, L. V., & Olkin, I. (2004). *The nation's report card evolution and perspectives*. Bloomington: Phi Delta Kappa Education Foundation.
38. Kolstad, A. (2006). *Basic Sampling Concepts Used in NAEP*. https://www.nagb.gov/content/dam/nagb/en/documents/naep/kolstad-sampling.pdf

39. von Davier, M., Sinharay, S., Oranje, A., & Beaton, A. (2007). The statistical procedures used in National Assessment of Educational Progress: Recent developments and future directions. In C. R. Rao & S. Sinharary (Eds.), *Handbook of statistics* (Vol. 26, pp. 1039–1055). New York: Elsevier. https://doi.org/10.1016/S0169-7161(06)26032-2
40. Reilly, D., Neumann, D. L., & Andrews, G. (2015). Sex differences in mathematics and science: A meta-analysis of National Assessment of Educational Progress assessments. *Journal of Educational Psychology, 107*(3), 645–662. https://doi.org/10.1037/edu0000012
41. OECD. (2019). *Mathematics performance (PISA)*.https://data.oecd.org/pisa/mathematics-performance-pisa.htm#indicator-chart
42. OECD. (2019). *Reading performance (PISA)*. https://data.oecd.org/pisa/reading-performance-pisa.htm#indicator-chart
43. Machin, S., & Pekkarinen, T. (2008). Global sex differences in test score variability. *Science, 322*, 1331–1332. https://doi.org/10.1126/science.1162573
44. Machin, S., & Pekkarinen, T. (2008). Supporting Online Material for Global sex differences in test score variability. *Science, 322*, 1331–1332. https://doi.org/10.1126/science.1162573
45. TIMSS & PIRLS. (2023). https://timssandpirls.bc.edu/isc/publications.html
46. Neidorf, T. S., Binkley, M., Gattis, K., & Nohara, D. (2006). *Comparing Mathematics Content in the National Assessment of Educational Progress (NAEP), Trends in International Mathematics and Science Study (TIMSS), and Program for International Student Assessment (PISA) 2003 Assessments (NCES 2006-029)*. U.S. Department of Education. Washington, DC: National Center for Education Statistics. http://nces.ed.gov/pubsearch
47. Eells, W. C., & Fox, C. S. (1932). Sex differences in mathematical achievement of junior college students. *Journal of Educational Psychology, 23*, 381–386. https://doi.org/10.1037/h0072425
48. Gates, A. I. (1961). Sex differences in reading ability. *The Elementary School Journal, 61*, 431–434. https://doi.org/10.1086/459919
49. Flynn, J. M., & Rahbar, M. H. (1994). Prevalence of reading failure in boys compared with girls. *Psychology in the Schools, 31*, 66–71.
50. Logan, S., & Johnston, R. (2009). Gender differences in reading ability and attitudes: Examining where the differences lie. *Journal of Research in Reading, 32*(2), 199–214. https://doi.org/10.3318/dib.004314.v1
51. Robinson, N. M., Abbott, R. D., Berninger, V. W., & Busse, J. (1996). The structure of abilities in math-precocious young children: Gender similarities and differences. *Journal of Educational Psychology, 88*, 341–352. https://doi.org/10.1037/0022-0663.88.2.341
52. Svensson, A. (1971). *Relative achievement, school performance in relation to intelligence, sex and home environment*. Stockholm: Almquist & Wiksell.
53. Maccoby, E. E., & Jacklin, C. N. (1974). *The psychology of sex differences*. Stanford, CA: Stanford University Press. https://doi.org/10.1515/9781503620780
54. Mills, C. J., Ablard, K. E., & Stumpf, H. (1993). Gender differences in academically talented students' mathematical reasoning: Patterns across age and subskills. *Journal of Educational Psychology, 85*, 340–346. https://doi.org/10.1037/0022-0663.85.2.340
55. Benbow, C. P., & Stanley, J. C. (1980). Sex differences in mathematical ability: Fact or artifact? *Science, 210*, 1262–1264. https://doi.org/10.1126/science.7434028
56. Keating, D. P. (1976). Discovering quantitative precocity. In D. P. Keating (Ed.), *Intellectual talent: Research and development* (pp. 23–31). Baltimore: Johns Hopkins Press.
57. Kovas, Y., Haworth, C. M. A., Dale, P. S., & Plomin, R. (2007). The genetic and environmental origins of learning abilities and disabilities in the early school years. *Monographs of the Society for Research in Child Development, 72*(3), Serial No. 288. https://doi.org/10.1111/j.1540-5834.2007.00439.x
58. Chiu, M.-S. (2021). Gender differences in effects of father/mother parenting on mathematics achievement growth: A bioecological model of human development. *European Journal of Psychology of Education, 36*, 827–844. https://doi.org/10.1007/s10212-020-00506-0
59. Colmar, S., Liem, G. A. D., Connor, J., & Martin, A. J. (2019). Exploring the relationships between academic buoyancy, academic self-concept, and academic performance: A study of

mathematics and reading among primary school children. *Educational Psychology, 19*, 1068–1089. https://doi.org/10.1080/01443410.2019.1617409
60. Cascella, C. (2020). Intersectional effects of socioeconomic status, phase and gender mathematics achievement. *Educational Studies, 46*(4), 476–496. https://doi.org/10.1080/03055698.2019.1614432
61. Di Tommaso, M. L., Mendolia, S., & Contini, D. (2016). The gender gap in mathematics achievement: Evidence from Italian data. *IZA Discussion Paper, No. 10053*. Forschungsinstitut zur Zukunft der Arbeit (Institute for the Study of Labor). Bonn: Germany. https://doi.org/10.2139/ssrn.2810464
62. Ng'ang'a, A., Mureithi, L. P., & Wambugu, A. (2018). Mathematics gender gaps in Kenya: Are resource differentials between boys and girls to blame? *Cogent Education, 5*, 1564163. https://doi.org/10.1080/2331186X.2018.1564163
63. Mechanical calculator. (2021). In Wikipedia. https://en.wikipedia.org/wiki/Mechanical_calculator
64. Thorndike, E. L. (1907). *Empirical studies in theoretical measurements*. New York: Science Press.
65. Lincoln, A. E. (1927). *Sex differences in the growth of American school children*. Baltimore: Warwick & York.
66. Woolley, H. T. (1910). A review of the recent literature on the psychology of sex. *Psychological Bulletin, 7*(10), 335–342.
67. Woolley, H. T. (1914). The psychology of sex. *Psychological Bulletin, 11*(10), 353–379.
68. Judd, C. H. (1918). *Survey of the St. Louis Public Schools. Part One—Organization and administration*. New York: World Book Company.
69. Judd, C. H. (1918). *Survey of the St. Louis Public Schools. Part Two—The work of the schools*. New York: World Book Company.
70. Courtis, S. A. (1911–1912). The Courtis tests in arithmetic. *Committee on School Inquiry (1911–1913). Report of Committee on School Inquiry Board of Estimate and Apportionment, City of New York* (Vol. 1, pp. 389–546). City of New York. Republished by Forgotten Books, London.
71. Brooks, F. D. (1921). *Changes in mental traits with age: Determined by annual re-tests*. New York: Teachers College, Columbia University.
72. Thorndike, E. L. (1914). Measurements of ability to solve arithmetic problems. *Pedagogical Seminary, 21*(4), 495–503. https://doi.org/10.1080/08919402.1914.10534680
73. Shields, S. A. (1975). Functionalism, Darwinism, and the psychology of women. *American Psychologist, 30*(7), 741–754. https://doi.org/10.1037/h0076948
74. Hyde, J. S. (2005). The gender similarities hypothesis. *American Psychologist, 60*, 581–592. https://doi.org/10.1037/0003-066X.60.6.581
75. Mandler, G., & Kessen, W. (1959). *The language of psychology*. New York: Wiley.
76. Hellinger distance. (2022). In Wikipedia. https://en.wikipedia.org/wiki/Hellinger_distance
77. Shuster, J. J. (2021). Meta-Analysis 2020: A Dire Alert and a Fix. *Biostatistics and Biometrics, 10*(3), 555788. https://doi.org/10.19080/BBOAJ.2021.10.555788
78. Contini, D., Di Tommaso, M. L., & Mendolia, S. (2017). The gender gap in mathematics achievement: Evidence from Italian data. *Economics of Education Review, 58*, 32–42. https://doi.org/10.1016/j.econedurev.2017.03.001
79. Gallagher, A. M., & Kaufman, J. C. (Eds.) (2005). *Gender differences in mathematics: An integrative psychological approach*. New York: Cambridge University Press. https://doi.org/10.1017/CBO9780511614446
80. Davies, P. G., & Spencer, S. J. (2004). The gender-gap artifact. In A. M. Gallager & J. C. Kaufman (Eds.), *Gender differences in mathematics* (pp. 172–188). New York: Cambridge University Press. https://doi.org/10.1046/j.1529-8817.2004.00098.x
81. Pansu, P., Régner, I., Max, S., Colé, P., Nezlek, J. B., & Pascal, H. (2016). A burden for the boys: Evidence of stereotypic threat in boys' reading performance. *Journal of Experimental Social Psychology, 65*, 26–30. https://doi.org/10.1007/978-3-319-28099-82255-1

82. Flore, P. C., & Wicherts, J. M. (2015). Does stereotype threat influence performance of girls in stereotyped domains? A meta-analysis. *Journal of School Psychology, 53*, 25–44. https://doi.org/10.1016/j.jsp.2014.10.002
83. Caplan, J. B., & Caplan, P. J. (2005). The pervasive search for sex differences in mathematics ability. In A. N. Gallagher & J. C. Kaufman (Eds.), *Gender differences in mathematics* (pp. 25–47). Cambridge University Press: New York. https://doi.org/10.1017/CBO9780511614446.003
84. Ceci, S. J., Williams, W. W., & Barnett, S. M. (2009). Women's underrepresentation in science: Sociocultural and biological considerations. *Psychological Bulletin, 135*(2), 218–261. https://doi.org/10.1037/a0014412
85. Ceci, S. J., Williams, W. W., & Barnett, S. M. (2009). Supplemental materials. https://doi.org/10.1037/a0014412.supp
86. Dobyns, W. B., Filauro, A., Tomson, B. N., Chan, A. S., Ho, A. W., Ting, N. T., et al. (2004). Inheritance of most X-linked traits is not dominant or recessive, just X-linked. *American Journal of Medical Genetics, 129A*, 136–143. https://doi.org/10.1002/ajmg.a.30123.PMID.15316978
87. Fine, C., Dupre, J., & Joel, D. (2017). Sex-linked behavior, evolution, stability, and variability. *Trends in Cognitive Sciences, 21*(9), 666–673. https://doi.org/10.1016/j.tics.2017.06.012
88. O'Connor, J. (1943). *Structural visualization*. Boston: Human Engineering Laboratory.
89. Boles, D. D. (1980). X-linkage of spatial ability: A critical review. *Child Development, 51*, 625–635. https://doi.org/10.2307/1129448
90. Bouchard, T. J., & McGee, M. G. (1977). Sex differences in human spatial ability: Not an X-linked recessive gene effect. *Social Biology, 24*, 332–335. https://doi.org/10.1080/19485565.1977.9988304
91. Thomas, H. (1983). Familial correlational analyses, sex differences, and the X-linked gene hypothesis. *Psychological Bulletin, 93*, 427–440. https://doi.org/10.1037/0033-2909.93.3.427
92. Brick, C., Hood, B., Ekrol, V., & de-Wit, L. (2022). Illusory essences: A bias holding back theorizing in psychological science. *Perspectives on Psychological Science, 17*(2), 491–506. https://doi.org/10.1177/1745691621991838
93. Pinson, A., Xing, L., Namba, T., Kalebic, N., Peters, J., Oegema, C. E., et al. (2022). Human TKTL1 implies greater neurogenesis in frontal neocortex of modern humans than Neanderthals. *Science, 377*, eabl6422. https://doi.org/10.1126/science.abl6422
94. Box, J. F. (1979). *R. A. Fisher, The life of a scientist*. New York: Wiley.
95. Fisher, R. A. (1958). *The genetical theory of natural selection* (2nd ed.). New York: Dover.
96. Ellegren, H. (2011). Sex-chromosome evolution: Recent progress in and the influence of male and female heterogamety. *Nature Reviews: Genetics, 12*, 157–166. https://doi.org/10.1038/nrg2948
97. Zohar, A. H. (1990) *Mathematical reasoning ability: Its structure and some aspects of its genetic transmission*. Doctoral dissertation, Hebrew University, Jerusalem.
98. Thomas, H., & Jamison, W. (1981). A test of the X-linked genetic hypothesis for sex differences on Piaget's water-level task. *Developmental Review, 1*, 274–283. https://doi.org/10.1016/0273-2297(81)90022-8
99. Thomas, H., & Lohaus, A. (1993). *Modeling growth and individual differences in spatial tasks*. Chicago: University of Chicago Press. *Monographs of the Society for Research in Child Development, 58*(9), Serial 237.https://doi.org/10.2307/1166121
100. Thomas, H., & Kail, R. (1991). Sex differences in speed of mental rotation and the X-linked genetic hypothesis. *Intelligence, 115*, 17–32. https://doi.org/10.1016/0160-2896(91)90020-E
101. Johnson, W., Carothers, A., & Deary, I. J. (2009). A role for the X chromosome in sex differences in variability in general intelligence? *Perspectives in Psychological Science, 4*, 598–611. https://doi.org/10.1111/j.1745-6924.2009.01168.x
102. Turkheimer, E. L., & Halpern, D. F. (2009). Sex differences in variability for cognitive measures: Do the ends justify the genes? (Commentary on Johnson et al., 2009). *Perspectives in Psychological Science, 4*(6), 612–614. https://doi.org/10.1111/j.1745-6924.2009.01169.x

103. Thomas, H. (1982). A strong developmental theory of field dependence independence. *Journal of Mathematical Psychology, 26*, 169–178. https://doi.org/10.1016/0022-2496(82)90041-4
104. Thomas, H. (1985). A theory of high mathematical aptitude. *Journal of Mathematical Psychology, 29*, 231–242. https://doi.org/10.1016/0022-2496(85)90016-1
105. Berletch, J. B., Yang, F., Xu, J., Carrel, L., & Disteche, C. M. (2011). Genes that escape from X inactivation. *Human Genetics, 130*, 237–245. https://doi.org/10.1007/s00439-011-1011-z
106. Craig, I. W., Harper, E., & Loat, C. S. (2004). The genetic basis for sex differences in human behaviour: Role of sex chromosomes. *Annals of Human Genetics, 68*, 269–284. https://doi.org/10.1046/j.1529-8817.2004.00098.x
107. Wang, P. J., McCarrey, J. R., Yang, F., & Pagel, D. C. (2001). An abundance of X-linked genes expressed in spermatogonia. *Nature Genetics, 27*, 422–426. https://doi.org/10.1038/86927
108. Zechner, U., Wilda, M., Keher-Sawatzki, H., Vogel, W., Fundele, R., & Hameister, H. (2001). A high density of X-linked genes for general cognitive ability: A run-away process for shaping human evolution? *Trends in Genetics, 17*(12), 697–701. https://doi.org/10.1016/S0168-9525(01)02446-5
109. OMIM. (2021). Online Mendelian Inheritance in Man. https://omim.org
110. R Core Team. (2020). *R: A language and environment for statistical computing*. R Foundation for Statistical Computing, Vienna, Austria. https://www.R-project.org
111. Lewis, J. C., & Hoover, H. D. (1987). Differential prediction of academic achievement in elementary and junior high school by sex. *Journal of Early Adolescence, 7*, 107–115. https://doi.org/10.1177/0272431687071009
112. Committee Final Report. (1911–1913). *School inquiry board of estimate and apportionment presenting summary of conclusions of the inquiry conducted by the committee*. City of New York. Republished by Hard Press Publishing, Miami FL.
113. Courtis, S. A. (1909). Measurement of growth and efficiency in arithmetic. *The Elementary School Teacher, 10*(2), 58–74.
114. Courtis, S. A. (1909). Measurement of growth and efficiency in arithmetic. *The Elementary School Teacher (continued), 10*(4), 177–199.
115. Courtis, S. A. (1910). Measurement of growth and efficiency in arithmetic. *The Elementary School Teacher (continued), 11*(4), 171–185.
116. Courtis, S. A. (1911). Measurement of growth and efficiency in arithmetic. *The Elementary School Teacher (continued), 11*(7), 360–370.
117. Courtis, S. A. (1911). Measurement of growth and efficiency in arithmetic. *The Elementary School Teacher (continued), 11*(10), 528–538.
118. Curry, A. (2023). Ancient DNA upends European prehistory. *Science, 379*, 865–866. https://doi.org/10.1126/science.adh3912
119. Posth, C., Yu, H., Ghalichi, A., Rougier, H., Crevecoeur, I., Huang, Y., et al. (2023). Palaeogenomics of Upper Palaeolithic to Neolithic European hunter-gatherers. *Nature, 615*, 117–126. https://doi.org/10.1038/s41586-023-05726-0
120. Humphreys, K., Grankvist, A., Leu, M., Hall, P., Liu, J., et al. (2011). The genetic structure of the Swedish population. *PLoS ONE, 6*(8), e22547. https://doi.org/10.1371/journal.pone.0022547
121. Makel, M. C., Wai, J., Peairs, K., & Putallaz, M. (2016). Sex differences in the right tail of cognitive abilities: An update and cross-cultural extension. *Intelligence, 59*, 8–15. https://doi.org/10.1016/j.intell.2016.09.003
122. Stoet, G., & Geary, D. C. (2013). Sex differences in mathematics and reading achievement are inversely related: Within-and across-nation assessment of 10 years of PISA data. *PLOS ONE, 8*(3), 1–10. https://doi.org/10.1371/journal.pone.0057988
123. Devlin, K. (2001). *The Math Gene: How mathematical thinking evolved and why numbers are like gossip*. New York: Basic Books.
124. Roy, M.-F., Guillopé, C., Cesa, M., Ivie, R., White, S., Mihaljevic, H., et al. (2020). *Global approach to the gender gap in mathematical, computing, and natural sciences: How to measure it, how to reduce it?* https://doi.org/10.5281/zenodo.3882609

125. Box, G. E. P. (1976). Science and statistics. *Journal of the American Statistical Association, 71*, 791–799. https://doi.org/10.1080/01621459.1976.10480949
126. Archer, J. (2006). The importance of theory for evaluating evidence on sex differences. *American Psychologist, 61*(6), 638–639. https://doi.org/10.1037/003-066X.61.6.638
127. Ritchie, S. J., Cox, S. R., Xueyi, S., Lombardo, M. V., Reus, L. M., Alloza, C., et al. (2018). Sex differences in the adult human brain: Evidence from 5216 UK Biobank participants. *Cerebral Cortex, 28*, 2959–2975. https://doi.org/10.1093/cercor/bhy109
128. Thomas, H. (1996). Between sex differences are often averaging artifacts. *Behavior & Brain Sciences, 19*(2), 265. https://doi.org/10.1017/S0140525X00042631
129. Everitt, B. S., & Hand, D. J. (1981). *Finite mixture distributions*. London: Chapman & Hall. https://doi.org/10.1007/978-94-009-5897-5
130. Thomas, H. (1993). A theory explaining sex differences in high mathematical ability has been around for some time (Commentary). *Behavioral & Brain Sciences, 16*, 187–190. https://doi.org/10.1017/s0140525x00029575
131. Spelke, E. S. (2005). Sex differences in intrinsic aptitude for mathematics and science? A critical review. *American Psychologist, 60*, 950–958. https://doi.org/10.1037/0003-066X.60.9.950
132. Penner, A. M. (2008). Gender differences in extreme mathematical achievement: An international perspective on biological and social factors. *American Journal of Sociology, 114*(Supplement), S138–S170. https://doi.org/10.1086/589252
133. Average human height by country. (2023). In Wikipedia. https://en.wikipedia.org/wiki/Average_human_height_by_country
134. Eisenberg, D. T. A., Kuzawa, C. W., & Hayes, M. G. (2010). Worldwide Allele frequencies of the human Apolipoprotein E gene: Climate, local adaptations, and evolutionary history. *American Journal of Physical Anthropology, 143*, 100–111. https://doi.org/10.1002/ajpa.21298
135. Günther, T., & Jakobsson, M. (2016). Genes mirror migration cultures in prehistoric Europe—A population genomic perspective. *Current Opinion in Genetics & Development, 41*, 115–123. https://doi.org/10.1016/j.gde.2016.09.004
136. Menozzia, P., Piazza, A., & Cavalli-Sforza, L. (1978). Synthetic maps of human gene frequencies in Europeans. *Science, 201*, 786–792. https://doi.org/10.1126/science.356262
137. Wang, H., Yang, M., Wandue, S., Lu, H., Chen, H., Li, L., et al. (2023). Human genetic history on the Tibetan Plateau in the past 5100 years. *Science Advances, 9*, eadd5582. https://doi.org/10.1126/sciadv.add5582
138. Young, A. I., Benonisdottir, S., Przeworski, M., & Kong, A. (2019). Deconstructing the sources of genotype-phenotype associations in humans. *Science, 365*, 1396–1400. https://doi.org/10.1126/Science.aax3710
139. Abell, N. S., DeGorter, M. K., Gloudemans, M. J., Greenwald, E., Smith, K. S., Zihuai, H., et al. (2022). Multiple causal variants underlie genetic associations in humans. *Science, 375*(6586), 1247–1254. https://doi.org/10.1126/Science.abj5117
140. Plomin, R., & von Stumm, S. (2018). The new genetics of intelligence. *Nature Reviews Genetics, 19*(3), 148–159. https://doi.org/10.1038/nrg.2017.104
141. Charney, E. (2022). The "Golden Age" in behavior genetics? *Perspectives on Psychological Science*, 1–23. https://doi.org/10.1177/17456916211041602
142. Schacherer, J. (2016). Beyond the simplicity of Mendelian inheritance. *C. R. Biologies, 339*, 284–288. https://doi.org/10.1016/j.crvi.2016.04.006
143. Finn, E. H., & Misteli, T. (2019). Molecular basis and biological function of variability in spatial genome organization. *Science, 365*, eaaw9498. https://doi.org/10.1126/science.aaw9498
144. Wai, J., Cacchio, M., Putallaz, M., & Makel, M. C. (2010). Sex differences in the right tail of cognitive abilities: A 30 year examination. *Intelligence, 38*, 412–423. https://doi.org/10.1016/j.intell.2010.04.006

145. Bahar, A. K. (2021). Trends in gender disparities among high-achieving students in mathematics: An analysis of the American Mathematics Competition (AMC). *Gifted Child Quarterly, 65*(2), 167–184. https://doi.org/10.1177/0016986220960453
146. Bradley, E. L. (1985). Overlapping coefficient. In S. Kotz & N. L. Johnson (Eds.), *Encyclopedia of statistical science* (Vol. 6, pp. 546–547). New York: Wiley.
147. Marks, G. N. (2008). Accounting for the gender gaps in student performance in reading and mathematics: Evidence from 31 countries. *Oxford Review of Education, 34*, 89–109. https://doi.org/10.1080/03054980701565279
148. Breda, T., & Napp, C. (2019). Girls' comparative advantage in reading can largely explain the gender gap in math-related fields. *Proceedings National Academy of Sciences, 116*(31), 15435–15440. https://doi.org/10.1073/pnas.1905779116
149. Global Gender Gap Report. (2022). In Wikipedia. https://en.wikipedia.org/wiki/Global_Gender_Gap_Report
150. World Economic Form. (2022). *The global gender gap report 2022*. Geneva: World Economic Forum. https://www3.weforum.org/docs/WEFGGGR2022.pdf
151. Guiso, L., Monte, F., Sapienza, P., & Zingales, L. (2008). Culture, gender, and math. *Science, 320*, 1164–1165. https://doi.org/10.1126/science.1154094
152. Ireson, G. (2017). Gender achievement and social, political and economic equality: A European perspective. *Educational Studies, 43*(1), 40–50. https://doi.org/10.1080/03055698.2016.1237868
153. Stoet, G., & Geary, D. C. (2018). The gender-equality paradox in science, technology, engineering, and mathematics education. *Psychological Science, 29*, 581–593. https://doi.org/10.1177/0956797617741719
154. Breda, T., Jouini, E., Napp, C., & Thebault, G. (2020). Supplementary Information for Gender stereotypes can explain the gender-equality paradox. https://doi.org/10.1073/pnas.2008704117
155. Breda, T., Jouini, E., Napp, C., & Thebault, G. (2020). Gender stereotypes can explain the gender-equality paradox. *Proceedings National Academy of Sciences, 117*(49), 31063–31069. https://doi.org/10.1073/pnas.2008704117
156. Hill, C., Corbett, C., & St. Rose, A. (2010). *Why so few? Women in science, technology, engineering, and mathematics*. Washington, DC: AAUW.

Index

H. Thomas, *Sex Differences in Reading and Math Test Scores of Children*,
Monographs in the Psychology of Education,
https://doi.org/10.1007/978-3-031-41272-1

MIX
Papier aus verantwortungsvollen Quellen
Paper from responsible sources
FSC® C105338

FSC
www.fsc.org

If you have any concerns about our products,
you can contact us on
ProductSafety@springernature.com

In case Publisher is established outside the EU,
the EU authorized representative is:
Springer Nature Customer Service Center GmbH
Europaplatz 3, 69115 Heidelberg, Germany

Printed by Libri Plureos GmbH
in Hamburg, Germany